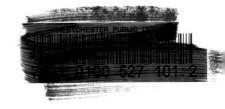

re·plen·ish

1. To make complete
2. To inspire or nourish
3. To become full again

# Replenish

### Experience Radiant Calm and True Vitality
### In Your Everyday Life

## Lisa Grace Byrne, MPH

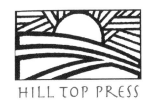

HILL TOP PRESS

ISBN-13: 978-0615855981

1st Edition, August 2013

Lisa Grace Byrne, MPH CHHC
Founder, WellGrounded Life
Web: www.WellGroundedLife.com
Email: Team@wellgroundedlife.com

# Get Instant Access to the Replenish Virtual Bonuses!

Go to:

www.WellGroundedLife.com/ReplenishBonus
and download them today.

This book is dedicated to my solar system:

To Jackson, my sun—
Madelyn, my moon—
and Brian, all my stars …

and to Michael, my center of gravity …
thank you for keeping our whole family knit together
in your strong and loving care.

And to the One from whom all good things come,
whose love sustains me every moment of every day.

# Contents

# Introduction

I'll never forget one of my first coaching calls. It was a lively conversation with a smart, funny, energetic mom named Laura. Our chatter was friendly and active, so I had to force myself to practice the art of the awkward silence. You know the unnerving pause that's the hallmark of therapists? Well, that's where I found myself on this call with Laura. Some bolt of wisdom struck me silent. I knew while our conversation was good, what was being said wasn't nailing the deeper issue going on. We kept skimming the polite surface, and so I waited.

And we endured the pause.

Until she blurted out, "I love being a mother. I just hate living the life of a mother sometimes." We both let out a collective sigh and teared up together. Now the silence we sat in felt warm and welcome. The truth right under the surface that was so hard to admit was said. That was the heart of the matter. Now that it'd been spoken without shame or judgment, but with complete and utter connection, now we could begin the work of steering her life in a different direction. One in which she truly did love being a mother and loved living out her life as a mother as well.

## Our Secret Conversations

Most moms I know feel brought to their knees in gratitude and love for the gift of motherhood. For the opportunity to be alive in a time when there are so many opportunities available, so many ways we can express ourselves and so many chances to squeeze the juice out of this incredible life. We wouldn't trade this role for the world, and yet, many of us are not experiencing it the way we want to be. We don't have the reserves of inner calm, we don't feel ready for our days with energy and vitality, and we don't know how to keep ourselves replenished *while* we're pouring out our lives for those we love the most. It's a paradox that leaves us feeling like we're wasting the most precious and amazing years of our motherhood journeys feeling depleted, scattered and flat. And we don't know how to change the direction we're heading.

I want to talk to you about a topic most of us don't really talk about … at least not in earnest with each other. There's a quiet, pervasive sadness I hear from women when they are brave enough to share their innermost experiences of the day to day life of a mother. It sounds like this:

- "Everything drains me; from the moment I wake up to the moment I go to sleep … there's just no joy left."
- "Somewhere along the way, I lost the 'me' inside. I know I'm a different person than I was before—I just have no idea how to get to know myself again."
- "I don't have a spare moment in my day. I'm constantly pulled in one direction and another – from my kids' needs to my husband's needs to the household needs, to work's needs. There is nothing left."
- "I give it all away – there is nothing left for me."
- "Most days, I'm just putting out the fires as they ignite."

When I hear these "secret" conversations from other moms, it triggers my own memories of when I felt exactly like that—when

I felt all my life energy was drained from the core. When the idea of energy, calm, and vitality felt laughable and triggered more cynicism than anything else in me.

But my life's different now. I used to feel I had to justify that statement so as not to come off like a snob or un-relatable, but I'm getting over that because I don't want the badge of living off fumes any longer. I wanted a different life. I wanted to live from a full and replenished well. I wanted motherhood not martyrdom. So when I say my life is different now, it is from a place of humility and gratitude. I made some honest assessments. I refused to define how things could be by what I saw everyone else doing. I decided I was going to define for myself what I really wanted out of life. Or, to be more accurate, I'm in the re-defining. I'm in the process of re-scripting. I'm learning to replenish while I'm pouring myself out day after day. I'm living in the paradox where taking care of your own core essentials opens up the capacity to give so much more of yourself to those you love.

I was reading an article a while ago titled, "Drowning Doesn't Look Like Drowning."[1] Its point was most of us have no idea what the true signs of drowning look like. Written by Mario Vittone, a Coast Guard officer, I was stunned to learn that over half of the children every year who die from drowning do so within twenty-five yards of a parent or adult. We have this idea that drowning is a loud and dramatic scene, but the truth is drowning is a "deceptively quiet event." I thought about this message for a long while. So often people are drowning in their lives and it doesn't look like it—not from the outside. There may be people in your life, living under the same roof, who have absolutely no idea what's happening inside you. I felt like this for the first few years of motherhood. It's devastating to feel as though your life is going un-witnessed, that what's happening under the surface is unseen.

# Get Out of the Water

C. S. Lewis was once quoted as saying, "When you see a man who's drowning, don't stand on the shore and yell to him instructions on how to swim. First get him out of the water. Then, later, perhaps you can teach him how to swim." For me, my drowning point happened when shortly after my second child, Madelyn, was born, though the seeds of depression were sown well before her actual birth. All the while I was pregnant with her, I was teaching high school chemistry part time, studying to become a certified holistic health counselor, raising a toddler, fixing up our home to put on market, and searching for a rental. I was tapped out beyond anything I'd experienced before. When I look back on it now, it doesn't surprise me that I fell into a deep post-partum depression in those early months after she was born. At the time, of course, I internally blamed myself for not being grateful enough or strong enough to keep it all together. One of the biggest wounds we have collectively as mothers around depression is how often we blame ourselves while we are struggling with it. As I think back on how stretched thin and stressed out I had become, it makes perfect sense that my body would simply not have the capacity to keep me resilient and well. It's so much less an issue of blame than basic biology.

Well meaning people all around me kept trying to teach me to swim while I was drowning. There were so many good suggestions on what I should be doing—I just couldn't do anything. I was overwhelmed to the point I couldn't take even a small step forward. There were so many pieces of my life that needed attention; I didn't know what to focus on first. The turning point came when I got very sick. Three months after moving into our new home, a common respiratory cold ended up spreading into a significant upper respiratory illness ending in two double ear infections and such intense vertigo that if I opened my eyes and moved even an inch, my mind would spin so violently I'd throw up. I found myself on complete bed-rest for a week. Ironically, I had what I had fascinated about for years—a stretch of time to just rest. To lie down long enough to actually begin to unwind without anyone's needs vying for my attention.

I didn't expect to get it that way, but there I was—alternating between deep sleep, drowsiness (because of the narcotics) and times of lying awake processing where I was in life. Everything felt broken: my health, my stamina, my vitality, my emotional wellbeing, my mental clarity, my relationships. I was dried up from the core. Whenever I considered how to get it together and feel a little better, those thoughts became a magnifying glass reminding me of how badly I felt in life. I'd get into mental dialogues about how difficult life felt. But this time, after days of lying in bed some new ideas began to surface. When I thought about how everything felt broken, the new responses were, "Ok, then. If everything's broken, there's only one way to start to fix it. You have to start with the raw essentials. You have to get back to the very basics of what your body, mind, and spirit need to thrive and be well in the world and you have to start there. Get those filled first."

## Focus on Your Foundation and Build from There

Just like that I knew. I mean I seriously, deeply, clearly—without any grey areas or doubt—knew what needed to happen immediately. The way to begin caring for yourself when life feels utterly depleted is by getting out of the water safely, and then learning how to swim. Whether you feel like you're drowning, or feel like you're treading water day after day and getting more exhausted by the minute, the first step is to take care of the core essentials of your wellbeing. Nourish the very basic requirements of a vibrant body, mood, mind, and spirit. And what you need at the most elemental level is calm (in your mind), control (in your thoughts), nourishment (for your body), rest (that's restorative), movement (that's joyful), quiet (for your spirit) and connection (that feels true). In this book we'll explore the seven core essentials that get us out of the water and able to catch our breath again because they build up what we need on a foundational level for true wellness. Each core essential has simple starting places that make huge impacts, so we'll begin there.

I was sharing a few laughs with another mom in a coffee shop recently about the craziness of life with three kids' ages six and under. She said, "I feel like I live in the movie 'Groundhog Day' most of the time." I completely relate, because that's part of the season we're in—our days often look like mirror images of each other. But what if we changed the kind of day we have over and over? This isn't about checking out of the life you have so much as it's about living out your amazing life from a place of fullness and vitality. And the way we do that is from the inside out. Taking care of the core essentials of our wellbeing and letting the calm, clarity, and vitality radiate outward.

# Chapter 1

# The Paradoxes of Motherhood

After the birth of my first son, I could hardly talk about the experience. I didn't know how to share it, didn't know who to tell or even what to talk about. Instantly, I catapulted into the terrain of new motherhood and so much of this new world felt completely foreign. Life submerged under a haze. I lost my orientation in a sleep deprived stupor. Life started to feel like a long dark tunnel most days. Long stretches of murkiness were speckled with piercing moments of inexpressible joy and elation. The difficult parts felt deeper and more intense than I ever could have imagined and the breathtaking parts were brighter and more pure than I ever had known. It was like something within me splintered.

One part of me could bond and love my little one. Could nurture and nurse. Could hold and rock and nuzzle and breathe in all the sweetness and goodness of his little being. One part of me reveled in the miracle of this experience, another part of me began to drift away and feel disoriented. I was alternatively calm and present and then instantly overwhelmed with anxiety and processing layers of grief internally with no idea how to seek out help. Motherhood felt like a huge paradox to me. I had times of exquisite peace and transcendence nursing a newborn in the early morning and times feeling racked with stress dealing with colicky crying hours on end. I'd vacillate between a monk-like serenity and a mouse-like anxiety. I'd never felt so deeply connected to another human being before and, yet, never felt so desperately alone either. I'd never felt closer to my life's purpose and at the same time more insecure or empty.

And while internally there was a terrain of radical extremes, I learned quickly to maintain an even, measured outer image. That first year, outwardly, I looked as if I was hanging in there, but inwardly I was on the fast track to burn out and patterns of self neglect were steadily put in place. I had shifted into survival mode on many levels, and over time, that became my new norm. Somehow I was getting through the day. Outwardly I was doing what needed to get done. Inwardly, my landscape felt disconnected and dry.

I've noticed women, and mothers in particular, keep giving well past when their tanks are empty. Most of us have an amazing capacity to get done what needs to get done—even from a bone-dry place. I call it functional survival mode. I've seen mothers live with extreme adrenal burnout for years—their life energy just tapped out of them—but they're still getting the kids to school. They're still checking into work. They're still correcting homework and making dinner and doing the laundry. But here's the rub. The gifts we give are fundamentally different when given from a full well versus a dry tank. The gifts, themselves, are different. You show up differently in your life and in your relationships. You may still make dinner when you're walking around like a modern-day zombie stripped of your life spark—but I can guarantee you, you're not experiencing life like you're meant to. Everyone suffers when you don't take back control and become the nourished, strong, vibrant woman you were designed to be.

# Overwhelm Epidemic

There's an epidemic of overwhelmed and depleted mothers in our culture. And the way we're trying to resolve this crisis is through band aid treatments, outdated models of balance, and media imposed expectations of how mothers should feel and experience life. This model is driving us into the ground. At least, that's where I found myself early on.

And it's where I meet hundreds of women whom I teach through my courses. We love being mothers. But when we start not loving our lives as mothers, it's a wakeup call that we need take stock of what's working and what's not. Most of the time, it isn't that we'd change much about the details of our lives. We just yearn for the experience of living it fully alive with an abiding sense of inner calm rather than struggling through each day. To be clear, it isn't a Polly Anna version of mothering we're going for. We're not trying to avoid the realness of the journey, the hard parts, the irritating and challenging and downright maddening parts of raising and loving little beings into the world. But it's doing so from a full and vital and well place. It's having resiliency to ride the rapids with a sense of hopefulness, a bigger perspective that keeps us firmly rooted in the goodness and blessing and grace of it all. The road to the life we desire is the road to establishing deep anchors of wellness so we aren't so drastically tossed around when life gets stormy.

# Small Trickles from Many Hoses

Imagine a large empty pool. At the dry concrete bottom are brightly colored plastic balls. These plastic balls are how we experience our lives. Imagine they're our physical, emotional, mental, and spiritual wellbeing. Without any water in the pool, they may as well be as heavy as lead—stuck to the bottom of the pool. Now, imagine that all around the pool are garden hoses pointing inward toward the center of the pool. These hoses are our core essentials of wellbeing. All we really need are small trickles of water to be turned on and the pool will begin to fill. Turn on a few at a time and the pool fills faster. But here's the thing—regardless of which hose you turn on, all the balls will rise. That's how it is with our whole-person wellbeing. You may assume nourishing your body with calming foods only impacts your physical health, but it actually impacts all the parts of your wellbeing. We're not compartmentalized beings; our body, mood, mind, and spirit are all intricately connected.

So as you work through these core essentials, know that even turning on the hose a small trickle, one at a time, is going to elevate all the areas of your life. All the plastic balls begin to float, regardless of which hose you begin with. The point is simply to begin and one by one turn on the water little bits by little bits. Cumulatively, the small extensions of care you give yourself add up to enormous returns in how you experience your health and vitality. When I began to see my own wellbeing as something that needed filling up rather than perfecting, it opened a whole new grace-filled way of loving and caring for myself. In this book, we'll take each core essential in turn and explore how we can turn the hose on a little bit at a time. Remember, even a small trickle from each hose will fill the pool ... even to overflowing. Let's take a walk around the pool and get a quick overview of each core essential before we dive in.

## The Seven Core Essentials Overview

### Core Essential #1: Calm Mind

Stress is a funny thing. This world has stressors. Uncontrollable and undeniable. And yet, whether your body experiences stress or calm has nothing to do with the stressors of the world. Not really. Not exactly. In this core essential we'll understand how we were designed from the inside out to have both a stress response and a calm response. Most of us only have our stress buttons exposed, and everything from the TV morning news to the thought of making dinner pushes it all day long. In this core essential we'll learn how to find our calm button and how to bring in practices that consistently keep us in a calm state throughout our days.

## Core Essential #2: Sovereign Thoughts

How you think about what's happening around you is far more important to your wellbeing than what's actually happening around you. Your thoughts are the most direct and powerful source of internal stress in our modern culture, so learning to be in control of your thoughts is crucial for your highest wellbeing. In this core essential we'll explore how to change stressful thoughts into life-giving and affirmative thoughts which create within your mind an oasis of calm, composure, and peace.

## Core Essential #3: Nourished Body

Food is an intimate way we can nourish and nurture ourselves back to wholeness. We'll explore this powerful tool in the larger scope of what it means to have a healthy relationship with the food we eat. Where food is simply one of the many tools you have to take care of yourself—not the only one, not the elevated one…but a powerful one, all the same. Keeping good foods in our bodies makes a huge difference in how we handle the demands of our days. When food becomes a tool that responds to what our bodies, moods, and minds need, it also becomes a deeper way to trust and care for ourselves in our everyday lives.

## Core Essential #4: Restorative Rest

It's become commonplace for moms to walk around in a sleep deprived stupor, clinging to paper cups of coffee. But without restorative rest in our lives, we'll never feel the vitality and clarity we're meant to experience and need in order to mother well. Although the disruption of sleep is a very real part of mothering young children, many of us consistently deepen the wound by our lifestyle choices. When I got serious about being a better steward of getting the rest I needed—the impact was significant.

## Core Essential #5: Joyful Movement

Healthy movement, activity, exercise…whatever you call it, many women have a visceral reaction to the thought. We've grown up with years of painful memories of forcing our bodies to move in ways that felt hard, uncomfortable and boring. As mothers we can feel like we are moving all day long, but have lost any connection to delight or sensuality around how our bodies feel in the world. Reconnecting to joyful movement again is a crucial element of our whole-person wellbeing. Movement that feels spacious, enjoyable and fun supports vitality not only on a physical level, but on a mental and emotional level too. We'll take time to explore how to discover what joyful movement is to you and how to make it a regular part of your life.

## Core Essential #6: Anchored Quiet

Finding quiet in a very noisy world is not always easy, but it's imperative if we're going to experience true inner vitality. When we live, love and mother in the world with our spirits tethered to a deep anchor, we can weather the storms. We can find perspective and truth to keep us aligned. We have our northern star established. We carve out times of stillness and quiet that our minds need and our souls crave and experience replenishment from an internal spring within us.

## Core Essential #7: Authentic Connection

We were designed to live in community, to connect to one another and bear the journey of motherhood together. And yet, we're living more isolated and lonely than ever before. Seeking out life-giving, authentic relationships is crucial for our well being on every level. In this core essential we'll talk about the key relationships every woman needs in her inner circle, and how to seek them out, receive them and manage life when they aren't present yet.

# Chapter 2

# Calm Mind

Have you ever felt like your attempts at self care weren't making much of a difference in how replenished you actually felt on a daily basis?

When we think about our inner sacred core, like a reservoir of wellbeing within us, it makes sense to consider ways to turn on the hoses. But sometimes, before we can begin the refilling, we have to look at the size of the pool itself. When our inner cup is extremely shallow, we simply don't have the capacity to hold much of the goodness we want to bring into our lives. Stress makes for shallow wells within us. And sometimes our attempts at filling up when we are chronically stressed are like aiming a garden hose at a tea cup—we simply don't have the capacity to receive deep, lasting replenishment.

This hit home for me when I had a stretch of off the charts bad days with the kids. I told my husband I needed a break. I busted out a gift certificate I was holding onto for a massage, we coordinated schedules, and I booked the first one available. I remember the moment when I bolted through the door to my car on the way to the massage. The kids were in massive meltdown. Two were in tears arguing and our littlest had just pulled down the maple syrup and poured it all over himself (and the kitchen floor). I kissed Mike goodbye and split. The massage itself was glorious—all zen-like with soft music, warm sheets, and essential oils. I lingered with my lemon water afterward soaking up the calm and peacefulness. On the way home I felt sure I had effectively replenished the stores. I was serene and relaxed. My muscles felt open and limber. My forehead was smooth and my jaw was gently closed. I was in good shape.

I came in the door ready to relieve my partner, who'd been faring in the ring for the past hour and a half, but no sooner did I re-enter, I felt like ice-cold water was thrown on me. The kids screaming, the dog tracking mud all over the floor, the baby crying. Immediately I was in absolute inner code-red, clenching my jaw, rubbing my forehead, and wanting to cry myself. It felt like the massage was a colossal waste of time. I spent the next couple hours battling monkey-brain mental chatter that spun around how insane life felt and how hopeless it was to think I could ever feel calm and grounded again.

Later that evening when I was processing the day, it occurred to me that all I ever did was hit the pause button from time to time with a massage or a mani-pedi. It'd been a long time since I felt truly reset, when I felt a deeper capacity to handle the stresses of life as a result of the care I gave myself. I thought hard about the pattern of self-care I'd been putting into place. It seemed so many of my attempts at taking care of myself would only go so far, they only made short term differences in how I was actually coping day to day—precisely because I wasn't dealing with the root issues at hand. Chronic stress was diminishing my ability to recover and replenish throughout the day. If there's one practice that has radically changed every single area of my life, it's the practice of calm—and in particular the practice of having a calm mind.

Turning on the calm is the most effective way of turning off the stress. When I tried to tackle stress head on, it always won. When I began to learn ways to dismantle its stronghold from the back door approach and click on the calm switch from within, everything transformed. Once this became my first responder of self-care practices, it impacted every other part of my wellbeing, from how I felt emotionally, to how I maintained my ideal weight, to the intimacy in my marriage. This was a powerful core essential and it took me a long time to get clear on how to maximize the tools of calm for my highest benefit. But once I did, everything started to shift.

Establishing the core essential of a Calm Mind is a way to expose the reset button instead of the pause button. It's a way to get out of the water and get our feet on solid ground when we've been treading for far too long. We have a tendency to want to keep moving our hands and feet faster and faster just to keep our heads above water, when getting out of the water and catching our breath is far more effective in the long run. The magic of this core essential is we can practice it in the everyday hectic-ness of life. We can do these practices when we are in car lines, changing diapers, rushing to catch trains, meeting deadlines, on the phone, kissing boo-boos, and passing out on the couch.

Most of us feel like we're built to be stressed out, because it's what we've known most of our lives. From the moment we wake, our minds begin to race and feel anxious. We feel everything about life is stressful and it's hard to imagine going through a typical day from a grounded place of vibrant calm. But calm is actually what you were designed to experience. You were designed to radiate calm from within, and impact those around you … most especially your children, by first setting the tone of the environment from your own inner thermostat.

# Thermometer or Thermostat?

I saw a bumper sticker once that read, "Thermometers react to the temperature, thermostats control the temperature. Which are you?" It's a good question, right? It helped me see how crucial my emotional tone was to the temperature of my home. When Jackson, my oldest, triggers me with his behavior or attitude, I feel like I can become six years old again myself. This, of course, is just another way of saying I lose all capability of setting the emotional tone of the interaction and shift into reactionary mode. I simply want to lash back at him with the same behavior or attitude. Have you ever found yourself yelling at your child not to raise his voice at you? Even as I do it I feel so foolish, and yet, it's also a huge sign for me that I'm in a stuck stress state and need to shift myself into a calm before I can even hope to regain my composure.

Kids are expert thermometers. They receive the energy, tone, and "temperature" from those around them. In fact, they're constantly trying to figure out what they're supposed to do by watching, modeling, and exploring our reactions to the world and to them. Think about what happens when kids are in tense or anxiety filled situations. Or when they are tired or hungry or it is just too hot outside. They are receiving the temperature around them and simply reacting to that rising heat. They often need a lot of help and guidance from us to cool off because they can't do it themselves. It is in their nature to siphon from us the tone and energy of their worlds. Ever feel like kids suck you dry? Well, it's because they do literally. (And incidentally, that's their job.) They're feeding directly off of whomever is closest to them in their worlds.

One of the things I believe we're meant to do for our children is to help them develop and strengthen their internal locus of control, help them learn to replenish their stores and stay well and vital. But here's the thing—we as parents can't help them if we haven't crossed over from a thermometer to a thermostat. And for many adults, we weren't taught how to replenish and remain calm, particularly when we're in high stress situations.

That's when this gets sticky. Stress causes us to become reactionary. So the key to being a thermostat in today's stress-crazed culture is to learn how to maintain an inner calm amidst the storm. Trying to care for yourself while you're in full blown stress response was like my one hour massage break in the middle of pandemonium—and not just one stressful day, but after many weeks of unchecked stress. It's like throwing a small cup of water on a blazing fire. Technically it's helping, a little. But in the grand scheme of things it doesn't feel like it's done much at all. When you're coming from a place of high chronic stress—which, by definition, is exactly where you are if you're feeling overwhelmed and exhausted—bringing in the core essential practices of a Calm Mind will absolutely transform your life. These practices tap into what I call the "master calm switch." We all have a master calm switch, which is like a back-door way to instantly shift our brains into a calm state. So instead of turning off the stress, our strategy is going to be to turn on the calm. In effect, it does the same thing—calm on means stress off—but turning the calm on is a much easier and faster process than turning stress off, so we're starting from there.

## Master Calm Switch Strategies

Limbic calming techniques, which target the limbic part of your brain where your master calm switch is located, are like back door techniques to regaining your calm and deepening your capacity to be truly replenished. They're far more effective than trying to bulldoze your way through the front door with your thoughts. Once you're in the back door you can effortlessly turn the knob of the front door from within. And that's exactly the strategy we're going to employ. First get into the house (your limbic brain) and calm your whole system down. Then, in our next core essential we'll use our thoughts to reinforce calm and deepen it. Now, let's talk about five different master calm switches and how these can be woven into our everyday lives.

## Master Calm Switch #1: Breath

Your breath is one of your most elemental and powerful tools to create instant calm. When you breathe deeply into the lower lobes of your lungs, you send a signal to your limbic brain to inhibit stress-producing hormones and trigger relaxation throughout your whole body. Many nerves are connected from your limbic brain through all parts of your body. The longest nerve in the body, called the vagus nerve, begins in the limbic area of the brain and ends underneath your belly button where it explodes into millions of nerve endings. The heart and gut are two of the most important organs it connects to. When you do abdominal breathing, your breath fills the lower parts of your lungs and expands your diaphragm, in effect stimulating the millions of nerve endings in your gut. These nerves then send signals to your brain to release high concentrations of oxytocin. Oxytocin is known as the love hormone. It calms you down, relaxes you, and increases your desire for deep bonding and connection. When oxytocin is produced, stress-hormones are blocked and inhibited. You've effectively turned on the calm.

There are many techniques for deep breathing that are simple, fast, and effective …though you can simply get started right now, without any advanced training. Here's a basic way, The Simple Deep Nose Breath, to get the full benefit of calming breath. Find a comfortable chair that allows you to sit with straight posture. Put one hand on your belly and relax your shoulders, stomach, face, and eyes. Begin by breathing in through your nose for a count of four while softening your tummy and allowing space for your lungs to completely fill. Now breathe out calmly for another four counts as you release all the air in your lungs and feel your stomach retreat inward to help push the air out. Be sure to breathe through your nose—this is how you send your breath into the lower parts of your lungs. When we breathe through our mouths the air stops short at the top parts of our lungs instead. Experiment breathing both ways right now and feel where the air stops in your chest.

Another simple technique is the Alternate Nostril Breath. Assume the same comfortable position as explained above. Then take the middle finger and thumb of your right hand and lightly touch them to either side of your nose. Begin by slightly putting pressure on your left nostril so it closes shut and breathe through your right nostril to a slow count of four. Pause with full lungs for a moment as you switch your fingers releasing the left nostril and softly closing the right nostril. Now allow the air to exit your lungs through your left nostril. Breathe in now through your left nostril and when your lungs are full, pause, and switch nostrils again so the air can be released through the right nostril. Continue in this pattern for a few minutes.

Try to give yourself five minutes of deep breathing a few times a day—maybe once in the morning and once before bedtime to start. Set a timer and allow yourself to simply follow your breath in and out to simple counts of four until the five minutes are up.

## Master Calming Switch #2: Olfactory Nerve

At the very top, inner part of your nose sits the olfactory nerve. This is the nerve that recognizes and processes your sense of smell. We're able to register smells because molecules that have an aroma or scent are very small ring-like structures called aromatics. These very small molecules easily become airborne and we breath them in allowing them to hit our olfactory nerves. In nature, the strong aromas of plants and flowers all contain these aromatic molecules. Essential oils are the highly concentrated extracts of distilled plants, flowers, trees or shrubs and they have extremely high amounts of these aromatic molecules. When you take a drop of essential oil on your palm and breathe in the scent, these aromatic molecules rapidly vaporize and can be inhaled easily through your nose to the olfactory nerve.

Here's where the calming comes in. Your olfactory nerve is hard wired into your limbic brain. The limbic system, remember, is the emotional seat of your brain and controls heart rate, blood pressure, breathing, memory, stress levels, and hormone balance. Your sense of smell is the only sense that goes directly into this limbic area of your brain and can immediately stimulate it to shift into calm. There are certain essential oils that are particularly effective in bringing in relaxation, calming, balancing, focus, and invigoration through this limbic connection. Below is a beginner's guide to using essential oils as part of your calm mind toolbox. Simply take a drop (remember they are highly concentrated) of pure, therapeutic-grade essential oils in your palm. Rub your hands together, cup them over your nose and take a few deep breaths (and cash in on the deep breathing trigger while you're at it).

## A Beginner's Essential Oils Menu

*Relaxing and Calming: Lavender, Roman Chamomile*

*Cleansing: Cinnamon, Lemon, Basil, Oregano, Clove, Eucalyptus*

*Invigorating: Peppermint, Sandalwood, Lemon, Orange*

*Balancing: Cinnamon, Basil, Parsley*

*Uplifting: Rose, Bergamot, Geranium*

*Focusing: Cedarwood, Frankincense*

Another way to tap into the power of nature's aromatic molecules is to grow a simple herb garden on your kitchen windowsill. Herbs like Eucalyptus, Lavender, Chamomile, Peppermint and Basil are easy to grow and maintain. In addition to using them in cooking, you can take a couple leaves, crush them in your hands and breathe in their scent throughout the day.

## Master Calming Switch #3: Nervous System

Most of the time, when we think of stress, we think of the brain. But, the largest organ of your nervous system is your skin. When we soothe and detoxify our skin on a regular basis, we shift our nervous system into a calm response. When it comes to calming our minds through soothing our skin--think warmth and moisture. Things like warm baths and moisturizing with natural oils (bonus if you can warm the oils as well) are incredible master calming techniques. Your muscles, like your skin, are receptor organs which have the capacity to send calming messages to your central nervous system. Even giving your own neck, shoulders or feet a mini massage is very effective at turning on the limbic calm. One technique I love to end my day with is the hot towel scrub. It takes just about three minutes but puts me in an incredibly serene mood.

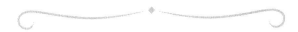

### *Hot Towel Scrub*

*You can utilize the exfoliating power in a simple washcloth. All you need is a sink that can hold very warm water, a washcloth, a few drops of essential oils or natural soap like Dr. Bronners liquid castile soap (my favorite is peppermint) and a few minutes alone in the bathroom.*

*Fill the sink with as warm of water as you can tolerate on your skin. The point is to feel the heat but certainly not to burn yourself. Then add a drop or two of essential oils or liquid natural soap. Take the washcloth, dip it in the water, and then ring it out fully. Take the warm cloth and begin to rub down each part of your body. You can begin with your legs, buttocks, lower back, stomach and side, arms, neck, face, and chest area. This is a deeply relaxing and restorative practice at the end of your day, especially if you struggle with difficulty sleeping.*

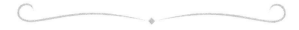

## Master Calming Switch #4: Energy

We all have physical bodies and energy bodies. In western cultures we're not as well versed with the nature of our energy body as eastern cultures that've studied and worked with energy healing for thousands of years, but nonetheless it doesn't change the fact that we have them! If you've ever had or seen an MRI, you've explored your energy body. Every cell of your body is made up of atoms. And every atom is made up of little moving parts called subatomic particles, like electrons and neutrons. Anything that moves releases a wave. And every wave has a frequency. So every cell of your body is emitting a frequency into the world. Now liver cells emit a different frequency than lung cells and so on. What the MRI machines receive are all the different frequencies from all the different parts of your body and chart your energies on a screen which coincides with all the different types of tissues you have. The fascinating thing is that a healthy cell emits a different frequency than an unhealthy or diseased cell, and so the MRI can also distinguish between a healthy cell and a diseased or cancerous cell.

I'm explaining all of this because it's important to take a little of the mystery out of understanding that you have energies running all through your body and out from your body, and that they're connected to your health and vibrancy. Remember all the parts of you are all connected, so when your energies are running low or sluggish it's often reflected not only in your body not working optimally but also your mood may reflect a down or depressed nature. It can be very powerful to engage calm and vitality through practices that keep your energies running optimally. A very dear friend of mine, Shelly, is a gifted Reiki master. When I have sessions with her my experience of calm is profound. Stress and fatigued adrenals will warp and jumble your energy flow. The energy patterns from a calm, vibrant body are different than from a stressed body. My work with Shelly keeps my energies aligned with the healthy patterns they're meant to be in. This is the power in working with your energetic body; it supports your highest health from a cellular level. Some energy healing techniques include Reiki, Qigong, acupuncture or acupressure, and reflexology. These are all wonderful ways to keep your body and mind well cared for. You can also learn energy techniques to do on yourself everyday to keep you in a high, healthy, frequency.

### *The Cross Over Energy Pattern*

*Here's an example of a very simple energy technique exercise I learned from Donna Eden[2] who's a pioneer in the energy medicine world. One of the ways healthy energy patterns move in our lives is through figure eights that move from one side of our bodies through our center and into the other side of our bodies. Draw a sideways figure eight in front of you that crosses all the way from your right side and to your left side making the little x in the middle at the center of your body. Anything that encourages a cross over pattern for your energy to flow is energizing and good for you. So a simple technique I use is the exaggerated march. This is especially good if I'm feeling in a funk. I'll begin my marching with raised knees and exaggerated arm swings where my right arm and right leg are both up at the same time. Then after a couple of marches I'll switch so I cross over and have my right arm up while my left knee is up and go on marching like this for about a minute. When I'm done I always feel lighter, more energized, and clearer. Resetting my energy flow in this simple way restores my calm response as well. A very fun practice to do with your kids, too!*

## Master Calming Switch #5:   Nature

Finally, the most powerful harmonizer I know of is nature. I can remember when I was dealing with Jackson's colicky crying night after night. The hours of un-soothable crying were so hard to bear I would ask everyone I met if they knew any tips to help. One older mom said to me, "Take a walk outside. When you feel you are going out of your skin, bundle yourself and your baby up and get outside. It may not end the crying, but it will help you. You'll be able to breathe again." And she was completely right. Sometimes it would calm him for a spell, but every time it would calm me—even a little, even under the intense duress of hours of crying and sleepless nights and depleted spirit. The fresh, crisp air, the large expanse of sky, the greens and browns and colors of the world soothed me and helped me feel connected to something bigger. We can start to believe our lives are very small and suffocating when we're indoors all day long. The simple act of getting outside and preferably into nature as much as possible is a balm. I've found it's crucial for a child's sense of calm to have a lot of outdoor time as well.

Even if you can't get outside in the moment, see if you can gaze at nature, or bring a bit of nature (like a houseplant, natural textures, an indoor waterfall, or even photos of beautiful natural settings) into your home as well. Researchers are coming to understand even small incremental exposures to nature act as powerful stress reducers in our lives. Studies show simply seeing a green landscape or stretch of trees through a window significantly improves your state of mind and calm response.[3] I have a favorite seat at my dining table that faces toward my lush and wooded backyard. Instinctively, when I need to unplug myself from a lot of high energy in the house, I'll take a glass of water and sit there, looking into the backyard and I feel significantly calmer.

I love rocks. I love collecting them, touching them, pilling them into cairns. I have them in jars all over my house. I remember an afternoon in the winter when cabin fever was causing us all to bounce off the walls. Between boredom, bickering kids, and a cranky mom, we were heading downhill fast. Then a jar of my rocks caught my eye. On a whim I took them down and sat on the living room rug. I began to lay them out in front of me and arrange them. Turning them over, noticing their colors and textures. Slowly the kids began to circle around me bringing their frenetic energy. So I explained mom wants to feel calm right now. If you feel like you can calm your energy we can all share and touch and look at the rocks together. You are responsible for your energy, if it gets out of hand; you have to choose to go somewhere else. They agreed (as much as toddlers can) and we circled around the spread out rocks. Soon we were all in bubbly conversation about which we liked most, what happens when you stack them, what colors we could find. I believe that having a connection to nature in that moment helped me set my internal temperature to calm. And from that place, we all had a much better chance of getting back on track.

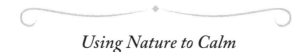

## *Using Nature to Calm*

- *Try to get outside every day.*

  *Whenever possible, choose to get outdoors when you start to feel stress rising. It can be tempting to hole away in the bathroom or bedroom when you have a small chance to reset, but when I take five minutes and get out for a few deep breaths or even a couple laps around the outside of my house, I always feel more renewed.*

- *Bring nature into your home.*

  *Each of our five senses is a gateway to tapping the limbic calm button in our brains. Consider bringing in nature's elements to your inner home environment. You could get creative with ways to look at natural textures in your home like plants, wood, rocks, sand, or shells. Bringing in small waterfalls or nature sounds on the stereo will engage your sense of hearing.*

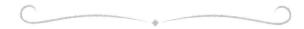

## Soften to Steady

I used to fantasize about being a perfect mother. I'd imagine what that would feel like, what it would look like. I'd go over scenarios in my mind around incidents when I felt like a major mom failure and try to envision how it would play out if I were just more put together, more in control of my own emotional reactions. In these imaginary scenes I'd never come undone.

I'd be solid, strong, and confident. I'd have instant access to clarity and wisdom on how to respond in every situation … what to say, how to act, the right answers, the wisest choices. I'd walk through life with unruffled feathers and my beautiful little ducklings would follow in cute wobbly lines behind me. Even the "messes" of my life would be tame, not at all like the ugly, tear-stained, guilt-inducing messes motherhood actually brought me through.

A hugely damaging belief we can hold is good mothers don't have bad days—really bad days. Good mothers don't get kicked off their horses- sometimes multiple times an hour. Good mothers don't have times of doubt and confusion around what to say or how to act as we raise these little people—almost all the time. The fastest way to crazy-making is to believe there's a way to insulate yourself from being knocked off center. No amount of self care, no amount of zen-like meditation, no amount of kale and whole grains, no amount of sleep or activity will keep you perfectly insulated from ever being triggered into a stressful state. And the truth, of course, is that trying to prevent yourself from ever feeling stressed is more likely to leave you heading toward code-red than anything else. The way to maintain a strong center of gravity is not to resist the tossing and turning, which is part of life, but paradoxically to soften into it. But softening isn't our first instinct.

It seems our first instinct is to stiffen and fight against the fall. In our backyard we have about an acre of oak trees. They have long and thin trunks; these beauties are sinewy and elegant. And when the wind comes, they sway. Watching them, I'm in awe they don't snap in two. The wind can bend them almost horizontal. When the pressure releases, they return upright and regal again. It's taken me so long to understand the paradox that it's better to soften rather than stiffen when riding the waves of an intense life with children. It's better to bend rather than break.

That's what the master calm switch techniques do for us on a daily basis when they're woven into the fabric of our days … they increase our flexibility even in the midst of challenging circumstances. And that's why they must be our first line of defense. Before we can master our mind, before we can use food as a nourishing tool, before we can truly find restorative rest, before we can silence the noise and receive the wisdom in stillness, before joyful movement or authentic connection … first we must learn to soften into the rocking and rolling waves of everyday life. We have to be able to shift gears when we're stuck in order to find a better way to move forward. And this softening is a shifting into calm. Stress will make you tense and tighten; calm will make you pliable and soft.

Before you move on, take inventory of these five pathways which tap into the master calm switch in your limbic brain. Jot down a few specific tools or practices you can bring into your life to support a Calm Mind throughout your days. Here's a quick summary of the tools we discussed.

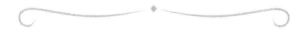

### Calm Mind Toolbox

- *Practice the Deep Nose Breath*
- *Practice the Alternate Nostril Breath*
- *Breathe in essential oils*
- *Breathe in aromatic herbs*
- *Take warm baths*
- *Moisturize with natural oils*
- *Give yourself a neck or foot massage*
- *Do the Hot Towel Scrub*

- *Do the Cross Over Energy Pattern Exercise*
- *Seek out support from energy practitioners*
- *Get outside everyday*
- *Bring nature into your home*

# Chapter 3

# Sovereign Thoughts

Meg is driving to pick up her daughter, Rachelle, who's at a friend's house. Her mind is already deep in an imaginary argument that began with her husband's sarcastic comment about her latest purchase before she left the house. She can feel her heart racing and a slight headache coming on. She gets a strong craving for a quick bite to eat. So she circles through a drive-through before arriving to pick up her daughter. Rachelle jumps in the car and starts to chatter about her day and Meg internally tells herself to stop stressing out and calm down. Hardly hearing Rachelle for most of the ride home, Meg is now fully absorbed in her own mind, trying to strong arm her stress into submission, and she's losing badly. For a moment, she comes back to the conversation with Rachelle just in time to hear her mention she forgot to give her teacher the form she was supposed to and ... Bam! Meg explodes and yells at Rachelle, who sits stunned, but then scowls angrily back from the outburst.

Oh wait, did I just say that was Meg and not me? Well, I'm sure it was Meg, too ... but it also sounds a whole lot like a pattern I've known in my own life. Swap out the details and I bet we've all come to a place where we knew we were reacting inappropriately but quite frankly we just couldn't get ourselves "unstuck" from the path we were barreling down.

## We Can't Start in Our Heads

We're stuck on stress. Modern life keeps our dials in the stress-on position. And the biggest source of turning on the stress switch is our thoughts. Though I know you're probably thinking, "No, Lisa, it isn't my thoughts, it's my tantruming toddler, it's the looming bills, it's the hours of mundane housework, it's the frantic rush of my schedule, it's my teenager wanting to date that guy …" Yes, our lives are full of intense and demanding (or even boring) times … but the truth is, the outer stresses of life must cross over a bridge in order to trigger an inner stress response within us. And that bridge is our thoughts.

Do you know someone in your life that doesn't care about being on time, it simply doesn't faze them? You may find that personality irritating, but it's not causing him or her stress. Because it isn't the deadline causing stress, it's how you feel and think about the deadline. Same with relationship stress. There are some people who do not have the same need for approval in order to feel good about themselves. They don't have deep triggers around that. Others of us find people-pleasing is as deep as our DNA and we stretch ourselves twisted trying to maintain pleasant and positive relationships. What's the difference? Our thoughts. When we believe something is stressful—through how we think or feel about it—it becomes stressful, physically.

But here's the rub, our thoughts can turn on stress, but they're very ineffective at turning off stress. So trying to think yourself calm isn't the easiest thing to do, at least when stress is already in the on position. Have you ever tried to talk yourself out of feeling stressed? Most times it's harder than brushing your toddler's teeth … and only makes you feel even more stressed-out. To turn the ship around, it takes a two-pronged strategy. That's why we explored the Calm Mind core essential first. Before you engage the tools we'll discuss in this chapter, remember to soften into calm first. From a limbic calm place, moving into the core essential of Sovereign Thoughts becomes much smoother.

## Melting the Polar Ice-Caps

We're going to talk about polar bears for a moment. Polar bears are magnificent creatures with some of the most advanced cold weather survival techniques of any animal on the earth. Living at the polar ice caps would require it. While many of us think of polar bears as white, they are actually black and white. Under the outer layer of white fur is an inner layer of black fur, close to the skin. Another characteristic about their fur is each hair is hollow and shaped like a cone.

See, in the arctic warmth is scarce. So the polar bear's whole body and biochemistry is designed to amplify the little warmth it has in its environment. When a ray of sun hits the polar bear's coat, the conical shape of its fur takes that sun wave and streams it down into the inner coat of fur. The inner coat of fur is black, and black pigment absorbs heat better than white, so the black fur, which is close to the skin, warms up. Now, when the heat from the black fur wants to radiate back out into the air, the outer white fur becomes like a glass pane and reflects the heat back down toward the polar bear's body. Fascinating stuff. And this is just one small example of the many ways polar bears were created to maximize the heat in their environment.

Now let's imagine that we transported a polar bear to the Sahara desert. The very same mechanisms that were crucial for the polar bear's survival in the arctic would now work against his survival in the desert. Now heat, which used to be scarce, is plentiful and the polar bear's design can't handle that.

Mamas, we're polar bears in the Sahara desert. Our bodies, physiologically and biochemically, were not designed to function properly under chronic, unrelenting stress. And I know you know this. I haven't met a woman yet who wasn't clear about the negative impacts of stress on her health. But I've been hard pressed to find many women who know how to consistently calm themselves and return from intense feelings of stress and depletion to a strong, calm and resilient place of living and loving again. In the modern world, our sources of warmth (our "suns" of stress) are often difficult to identify because they actually can't be seen. That's because a major source of stress for modern mothers is our thoughts. We trigger our stress response literally hundreds of times a day, not because our lives are in real danger, but because the stories we tell ourselves about our lives are stressful—and so our bodies respond that way.

When our minds are on spirals of negative stressful thoughts, we spend our days with an internal dial stuck on stress. Everything is impacted by it. It's like a colored lens—when we live our lives through the lens of chronic stress, it colors every single thing in our world. Alternatively, when we remove that lens, it clears and clarifies every single thing in our world. Becoming masters of our minds and generating sovereign thoughts provides massively powerful (and fast) transformations in our health and wellbeing.

## New but No Less Important

I remember a stretch of time when I found myself raising my voice and yelling at the kids more and more until it became apparent something wasn't working in how I was handling common situations with them. I felt absolutely sure that my yelling episodes were coming out of nowhere—in fact they surprised me because before I realized what I was doing, I was a full sentence into a high-pitched shout. What was most concerning was that these yelling episodes were not over anything major. They were the little annoyances, little pebbles in a typical day with kids that would find their way straight to the panic button within me. I kept asking myself "What is going on? What is the big deal? Why can't I just ride through these waves like a normal person?" I had fallen into a typical trap that most of us experience as new moms; I trivialized the new stressors in my life. I didn't even realize I had the potential to have such strong internal reactions to them. It was as if I looked at them somehow as "little stones," but because I wasn't acknowledging them they became a rock fall of tremendous weight on my mental and emotional health and I was getting crushed on a daily basis. From a bird's eye view, answering a question for the thousandth time, while a little tedious, didn't feel like something that my body should experience a full blown stress response over. But nonetheless, it could. After the thousandth "Mom" yelled out in need, I could feel my blood pressure rising. I would rub my forehead and squint my eyes as if I was in pain.

Part of the reason I ignored them is because they didn't look like triggers to me. I could feel myself tighten over things like the monotony, the boredom, the limits on my freedom, the dynamics around money and time within the context of my marriage, the laundry (oh God, the laundry), the physical neediness of children, and then the emotional neediness of children, the never-ending-ness of it. My new terrain was so full of these minor frustrations that I had worn down my own stress mechanisms and they were malfunctioning and sending me into major responses over minor things.

# The Super Mom Mantra

There were also the triggers around stories I would create in my own head. What I assumed others would think of me, what I assumed my mother thought of me, what my mother did think of me, what I thought I should be doing as a mom versus what I was actually doing, how I thought I should be feeling as a mom versus how I was actually feeling. If you aren't paying attention your triggers can start piling up like dust on the baseboards.

I was in the living room of the rental home one afternoon soon after we moved in. There were moving boxes scattered all around, in fact, I was semi-wedged between a couple boxes on the couch. I was nursing my newborn, Madelyn, and Jackson, my twenty-two month old toddler kept trying to climb on my lap with a book. I was jostling Madelyn to keep her positioned well while nursing and trying to reason with a not-yet-two year old about why I couldn't read to him right at that exact moment. It was such an unremarkable scene really. I had juggled more than this many times before, but this time, I cracked open. I broke down and began sobbing. All I could think was that I would never be enough. I would never be enough for everyone in my life. There would never be enough of me to go around. It was all just too much. I wanted out.

And that was really what I had kept trying to do from the very start of motherhood. I kept trying to be enough for everyone around me. Somehow I believed the ultimate purpose of motherhood was to complete and make whole all those around me. All the while, I was the one person who was becoming more and more incomplete and fragmented by the day. In the early parts of mothering, I set into motion an underlying pattern of how I was going to define my new identity as a mother. In its most simplistic terms, I was going to try to get it right. Not in the "I wanted to win a medal or badge because of it" way, but right in the "nothing in my life has ever felt more important to get right" way. Just the thought that I could possibly somehow mess this up and fail my children could send me to my knees. And the fact that it was an absolute certainty I was going to mess up along the way, a lot, left me a knotted, anxious mess. So without even knowing how to best judge what a "right" mother was, failing at this motherhood thing became fertile ground for all sorts of fears and insecurities to take root. It became fertile ground for misguided messages and influences to define who I should be and what I should do.

So much of my internal definition about mothering was guided by outside sources—and really, how could it not be? I'd never done this before. I had no idea how to define it from an internal place. I, like we all do, seek to figure out the unknown by trying to gather whatever information we can find about it. I found that my definitions of motherhood were sourced from so many places. What I saw my own mother do all my life, what I observed other mothers doing, what books and shows and websites and TV portrayed to me as a good mother. These definitions were all anchored outside of me. Many of the influences I wasn't even aware of but collectively they made up this vague but strong image in my psyche of a "good" mom.

Ultimately, I began defaulting to a definition that says a good mom does three things: she does everything herself, is everything to everyone, and keeps up the image that she's handling it all just fine.  We know logically this is an unrealistic definition, but I see moms all the time holding themselves to these kinds of expectations—I did for a while and the pressure drove me into the ground. When we try to do it all ourselves and be everything to everyone, we expend all our energy taking on everyone else's agenda and quickly lose sight of our own agendas. What's even more painful is that in order to be everything to everyone, we're often least to those who matter the most. I found the harder I tried to please everyone, the more often I was giving my family the worst of me. When we act as if everything is fine, it prevents us from showing up authentically; we become excellent image managers. Regardless of how bad I was feeling on the inside, I believed I had to keep up the facade that I could handle this and was doing great. The truth is, I never did this very well, but I berated myself internally that I must "look like a complete mess" to everyone around me.

Now to be sure, while I was caught in the web of this Super-Mom definition, I wouldn't have verbalized that I believed all these things. I would've denied that I believed this at all ... but my life and actions proved differently. Most of ours do. We say we don't believe we can do it all, but in the back of our minds we berate ourselves for not keeping it together. We have intense anxiety about asking for help. We keep our commitments even when we're falling apart at the seams because we don't want to burden anyone else or seem unreliable. We say we don't try to be everything to everyone, and yet we automatically say yes to every request, we overbook ourselves, we extend when we need to retreat, and at the end of the day, we reserved patience and empathy for perfect strangers while our children get our irritation and exasperation. We trudge forward, falling into a life of intense mental exhaustion. That three-pronged definition of motherhood nearly killed me. And I watch as it cripples mothers all over the place.

It cripples us because it becomes our foundational definition around what life is about. We can easily get hooked into believing that our job is to complete our children, when actually our job has always been and still is to complete ourselves. Your ultimate priority as a mother is wholeness, not perfection. Your job is not to complete your children. Your job is to complete yourself and then take that woman who's healthy, whole, and alive and show up as the mother of your children. When that woman shows up, she can make wiser choices and be more available to her children. This is the only parenting advice I've figured out so far. Do you want to know how to become the mother your child needs you to be? Become a whole and healthy woman. And take that vital woman and show up as the mother of your children. It's the only way. And a huge driver of stress in our lives is our negative, judgmental thoughts about ourselves.

## The Gift of Giving Meaning

One of the most powerful gifts we're given as human beings is the capacity to give meaning to our lives. To choose how we will define the events and experiences, the relationships, and the roles that we fill. When we define our lives, we have direct access to the sails. It's like tacking. When the winds blow out of control and cause the waves to be tossed like a washing machine, knowing how to shift the sails in response to the winds (or at times literally close them down) can steady the ship and keep it moving in the right direction even with tumultuous seas around you. Life has all the meaning that you give it. You have control of whether you access its highest meaning through how you think about your life and how you think about yourself. I know people who see miracles all over the place. I can remember after one of my summer trips to Africa, I spent three months feeling more free and joyful and alive than I had ever felt before. My days were spent with the mama farmers in the fields, in the huts, in the kitchens, in the hospitals, in the streets … learning how they lived, supporting them in what little ways I could, but mainly just being with them and sharing smiles and stories, sharing food and connection.

I'll never forget the one afternoon we were sitting in the shade of a tree in the middle of a field of beans. We all had piles of peas in front of us, shucking them and chatting a little. And then the small talk shifted among us into a bit of a hum here and there. Some women began singing a couple lines of a song to themselves and we all kept time in a loose, soft rhythm. When all of a sudden (at least to me, because I wasn't "in" on the slow hum thing going on, I was just a blissed out, content, happy little tag along, really), the whole group of these mamas started in on a massive chorus of a song. And the smiles spread like wild fire across their faces. They jumped to their feet in sync. A spontaneous dance party ensued—hands smacking, thighs making beats, dancing around, swaying, closing our eyes, arms up, and laughing. This is what joy does. This is what joy looks like when it sits and stirs among a group of women. It bubbles forth like a volcano and then in its right time settles down. After our happy explosion, we seemed to just naturally find ourselves on the ground again chirping away a little, back to shelling our beans. By most developed countries' standards, these women lived in poverty. But their minds were rich. They had a clear channel for joy, connection and happiness that I rarely see in my own culture. When I came home from that summer, something deep within me had changed. I understood how powerful calm, positive, and loving thoughts were to a life well-lived and well-enjoyed. I felt the world was in Technicolor. Everything shined to me, like from within. My life felt charmed. Indeed my life was charmed … just as it is now. Just as yours is.

While motherhood drove me deeper into truth and goodness and beauty, it also brought intensity and depression like I had never experienced before. It required me to relearn how to define my life with colors of joy, perspective, and hope. The difference is that after the laundry and the dishes, after the endless diapers and sleepless nights, after sore breasts and aching backs, after a body that's stretched and heavy, after low energy and a dull mind, after my days becoming others-focused and task oriented for so long, I saw the world more in shades of muted grays. A crucial part of becoming in control over your thoughts is learning how to rewrite your story in a truer, more positive, more grace-filled way. It's about wielding the powerful tool of our minds to right our ships—allowing our thoughts to be vessels of true replenishment instead of siphons of stress and depletion.

## Embracing the Paradox

Motherhood comes with everything—deep joy and deep grief, the good and the bad. Motherhood is full of paradoxes. Until we can accept that, it's difficult to move forward, to grow into our fullest selves. We get stuck in the angst of either/or thinking—either motherhood has to be this way or it has to be that way. What if it's both? By being honest about the paradoxes and holding them side by side, together, we can begin to accept motherhood for what it is. Saying one ("Mothering is exhausting and hard.") doesn't delete the other ("I love my children and feel incredibly blessed.") They're all my story—they're all parts of my journey. Our society and culture rarely provide space to hold paradoxes together and allow them to both exist. The messages tell us we have to accept one and reject the other. Author and blogger, Glennon Doyle Melton, says it this way, "I don't know how to make parenting easier, but I do know that it gets harder when we pretend it's not hard." Constantly pushing away our more difficult feelings about motherhood is exhausting. In my Vibrant Living Strategies workshop we begin by giving ourselves permission to tell our whole stories. All the paradoxes. We journal about the extremes we've felt on both sides of the spectrum. We open up about the gratitude, disappointment, joy, grief … all of it so we can put it out there, all jumbled together in one glorious mess and honor it for what it is—our truth, our story, our walk. Before we can make peace with our thoughts and turn our minds into refuges of calm within us, we have to stop fighting against the paradoxes we feel about motherhood and life.

Now, once you've given yourself permission fully to accept all the confusing, conflicting and undesirable feelings about your life … now's the time to take back the reigns and choose which story you'll focus on as you step forward creating the life you most desire. There is a difference between denying the whole spectrum of feelings and experiences we have and allowing ourselves to fixate and wallow in the perspectives that make us feel hopeless. Yes, motherhood is both hard and amazing, but which of these we choose to keep our mind focused on will determine the direction our life continues to go in. We can choose to draw from the colors on either side of the spectrum as we paint in the details of our lives. It's like going through an intense storm where you swallowed a lot of water and were tossed around. A bit later the sky clears, the sun returns, and you find your way to safe, solid ground. We can spend our time on the dry ground reliving the storm, or we can fill our thoughts with the promise of the dry land we're on now.

Once we relax into accepting all of the paradoxes, it's crucial to then make the choice of which perspective we'll choose to focus on as we move forward. And from that place we can begin the work of weeding out the thoughts that no longer serve us or are not true. Our next strategy in regaining the core essential of Sovereign Thoughts is about reversing the tendency for our thoughts to keep us in chronic stress and defeat, and instead turning our everyday thoughts into sources of life-giving honesty and refreshment, anchored in the truth about ourselves and our lives.

## Catch a Weed, Plant a Seed

For a while, I understood the general concept that thoughts could cause me stress, but I didn't exactly know how to identify them quickly. So it's probably a good place to start to explore what a stressful thought is and how you know a thought is a stressful weed in your garden. But first, an honest disclaimer. This process will feel like hard work, but we can do hard work and we can do hard things for the greater things in life. Think of all the effort people give in life only to receive the lesser things. I want great things for you and I want you to be equipped to pass on these tools to your children. The process gets easier the more you work it. It is like taking sandpaper to a very rough piece of wood. At first the rubbing is awkward and stunted. You don't feel like you are making much progress and you slip and get stuck. But every time you pick the sand paper up and work the wood again, it paves a smoother path. And once a little section becomes smooth the process gets exponentially easier and soon you are rubbing and sanding the wood with long, fluid, effortless strokes.

That's what this process feels like. It can feel rough and rocky. It can feel awkward and uncomfortable. You can feel like nothing is changing, but it is. Keep with it. Cover yourself with grace every single time you need it and get back up and do it again. The rewards are beyond what you can imagine when you live your life from a peace filled mind, with life-giving thoughts that anchor and nourish you even in the middle of a stress-crazed world. You become your own sweet oasis. Here's the four step process for catching a weed and planting a seed.

1. Catch a Weed: Notice and catch the stressful thought.
2. Plant a Seed: Restate the thought in present-tense, specific detail- plant a more true thought in its place.
3. Follow It Back: Follow the thought back to the core belief underneath it and test it.
4. Get Pro-Active: Is there an action step or a message to take away?

Before long, this process can happen fast and you'll work through these steps like one fluid movement. But in the beginning it is good to take it slow and take it step by step. At first, it was easiest for me to work through this process in a journal. When I started hearing a stressful thought going on repeat in my head, I'd note it down. As soon as I was able, I would take a couple minutes and put it through this process. After it goes through once, the next time it pops up you can move right through and weed it out quickly because you've already done the work. The best way to explain this is to illustrate it. So let's start with an example.

## Step 1: Catch a Weed.

The first step is to notice. In the beginning it was hugely helpful for me to learn some red flag words that indicated this was a thought I needed to weed out. The red flag words you'll want to begin looking for in your mental chatter are always and never. The problem with these words is they become like lenses. They're so generalized, they take a specific incident you are dealing with and color your whole horizon based on that specific situation. These thoughts are generalized like large umbrellas that cast darkness over your whole life. When your thoughts include "always or never," they are trying to act like core beliefs, something objectively true no matter what angle you look at it, something that you can count on to happen every single time.

Some examples could be: "My kids are always fighting," or "My kids never clean up after themselves," or "My husband is always judging me." Once you get good at identifying them, you'll be able to hear the generalized feel around certain thoughts and catch them as well. For example, you may think "It is impossible to go anywhere without a major tantrum." Do you hear how that statement is a blanket statement? While it doesn't have "always" or "never" in it, the feel of the statement infers it.   Step 1 is to catch the stressful thought. Once you hear it and identify it, name it as a stressful thought.

## Step 2: Plant a Seed

Step 2 is to immediately restate the thought in a truer, less generalized way using the present tense and specific details. So let's take the example, "My house is always a mess." Once that is caught as a stressful thought, we can restate it like this: "My house is a mess right now,"—or even better "The playroom is a mess right now." Many times when you get good at this process just this one step alleviates much of your anxiety. Stressful thoughts are like weeds because they can take over whole landscapes very quickly—and just like a weed in a garden, in our minds, stressful thoughts have a way of taking over whole dialogues for whole days. By restating the stressful thought, you pull it out and stop it from spreading. Once you feel or observe something in your environment that you're not happy about, you simply begin to state it in a specific, detail-oriented way and it stays contained.

So Step 2 is a simple re-write of the statement. Many times I'll even say this aloud to remind myself of what is really in front of me and to anchor in the process. In our example it becomes, "The play room is a wreck."

## Step 3: Follow It Back

Most of the time stressful thoughts feel stressful because of underlying beliefs we've attached to them. I've been programmed to believe that a home should be immaculate. That a clean home is a reflection on who I am as a mother. It's a different thing to want to have an orderly well-kept home versus connecting the state of your home to who you are and how you're adding up as a mother. This is where the journal work can be very powerful. Ask yourself, "Why is this so stressful to me?" Perhaps you explore:

"The play room is a wreck. The kids have not picked up their toys all day (or all week), that's not how I want my home to run. I want the kids to be more responsible for helping me keep the home neat and I could use better systems for keeping up with the clutter."

See how different that feels?

## Step 4: Get Pro-Active

Moving into Step 4, we consider if some action needs to happen to make things better. At this point, the solution is often clearer to see and less emotionally loaded. Maybe you decide, instead of having lunch right now, you're going to call a 1-2-3 clean up and get everyone's help to straighten up. Or maybe, your next step is simply to acknowledge the clutter with the toys is a major source of stress. You're going to consider ways you can create more order and have the kids more responsible for their share of clean up. The action steps will match what makes most sense for you, but they're empowered because they're based on the truth of the situation, not a loaded perspective that was tethered to an untrue core belief.

Stressful thoughts tend to make things more important than they truly are. Catching a stressful thought and disarming it is a powerful first step in generating the core essential of Sovereign Thoughts. In the beginning it'll feel like slow going progress. I have journal pages full of stressful thoughts being processed out, but the initial work pays in dividends when you begin to wield your thoughts easily through the day and truly become sovereign within your own mind again. Let's take a quick review of the tools we explored in establishing the core essential of Sovereign Thoughts.

# *Sovereign Thoughts Tool Box*

- *Challenge your definition of what a good mother is and does*
- *Embrace the paradoxes of your story and your feelings*
- *Choose which story you'll focus on as you move forward*
- *Catch a weed*
- *Identify your stressful thoughts*
- *Plant a seed*
- *Rewrite that thought in detailed present tense*
- *Follow it back*
- *Uncover core beliefs*
- *Get pro-active*
- *Make necessary changes*

# Chapter 4
# Nourished Body

The next core essential we'll explore is a Nourished Body—specifically how we nourish ourselves through the food we eat. Now eating food is something you do all day long, everyday. But, it's like a door you can open by either pushing forward or pulling backward. Depending on which direction you walk over the threshold, food can either bring you into a place of calm, clarity and vitality, or it can walk you straight into depletion, stress, and exhaustion. It's one of the most powerful ways we can establish a strong foundation of health—but it's a tricky one as well. Because, for most of us, food isn't a neutral tool. We have layers of emotional baggage woven into how we use food. When we have empty places in our inner lives, food can easily be used to stuff away the discomfort or boredom. We can eat to numb, escape, or distract ourselves. And so, while food has the potential to be a powerful way of caring for ourselves, many of us first need to understand the patterns and habits we have around eating before it can truly nourish us rather than harm us.

This is one of the reasons I teach about food in a different way than most of us are used to hearing about it. Instead of dissecting food into calories or grams and using it as a way to control ourselves, we'll embrace food as a way to respond and communicate with our bodies. When we start to use food as tool rather than a weapon, we unbind it from its emotional undertow and we're free to enjoy and nurture ourselves without guilt or restriction.

## Stress and Calm

For all the years and tens of thousands of dollars I've spent getting educated in the finer details of human nutrition, one simple concept has revolutionized my life: Food can either increase calm or increase stress in your body. Researchers in the world of nutritional biochemistry define these two different states in terms of inflammation.[4] When our bodies are calm and nourished there is very little evidence of systematic inflammation at the cellular level. If a specific area needs healing, you'll find inflammation there as the body's proper response. But overall, a healthy body is not an inflamed body. So when we feed our stress response, we increase inflammation and illness and perpetuate a stressed body and mind. And when we feed our calm response, we decrease inflammation and support calm, clarity, and vitality from the inside out.

Every moment, your biochemistry is functioning under either a stress response or calm response. Remember they are like a toggle switch— when one is on the other is off. And depending on which of these responses are triggered, everything can change. You digest food differently under a calm system versus a stressed system. Same goes with the capacity for you to do literally hundreds of other functions. You think, remember, focus, solve problems, uptake nutrients, regulate your heart-rate, ovulate, smell, hear, feel, taste … every possible way you experience life is done differently when you are in a stress state versus a calm state. Fundamentally, stress adds a layer of noise, chaos, and dysfunction to every system of your body.

When I found myself laid up in bed, sicker than I'd been in years, with an infant and toddler I could no longer care for, wondering how exactly I was going to start putting the pieces together again, I saw clearly and simply that if I couldn't learn how to shift myself back into a calm response, I was never going to change the direction I was heading. So as I wove into my life these core essentials, I wanted to figure out how I could use food to help my body and mind experience more steadiness and peace. This began a wholly different way for me to use food as a tool in my life. I began thinking of nourishing myself in terms of how I could calm myself. Seen in this way, food began to be stripped of all the dieting, emotional, restrictive, punitive layers it has been weighed down with in our culture. In not so sophisticated terms, I began asking myself, "What foods will deeply calm and nourish me right now?" And that has been my guiding question ever since.

Why does this works so well? Stress has to be fed, just like calm needs to be fed. When we're stressed, we crave certain kinds of foods. When we are calm we crave other kinds of food. I began to reorganize all the reams of nutrition information I had gained over the years and see foods as either stress-feeding or calm-feeding. The reason I believe this is so effective is it takes us out of the obsessive need to over calculate and get snagged in perfectionism around food. We are raised in a culture that is nuts around food. We were taught from very young ages to overanalyze our food in all sorts of ways—by calorie, protein grams, percent fat, and vitamin units. We've cheated ourselves from the true beauty and function of foods, and reduced eating to a controlled, restrictive ordeal.

## Another "Stress" Sun Is Sugar

It all comes down to this understanding: What was scarce is now abundant. Remember the polar bear example, where warmth was the thing that was scarce and is now abundant. We already talked about one "stress sun" in our lives as being our stressful thoughts. Another major "stress sun" is sugar. When you consider what food options we had before the Industrial Revolution, sources of sugar were few and far between. Sugar as a fuel source for our bodies was locked up in real foods with fiber and protein, fats, and nutrients—all which needed to be unpacked and digested before our body could utilize sugar for fuel. Your body needs healthy carbohydrates (which will convert to blood sugar through digestion)—in fact our brains can't run on anything else. But less than a hundred years ago, it was a rare commodity to have crystallized sugar. Before World War II, we didn't have the proliferation of chemicalized, artificial, sugared junk foods available to us now. The human body was never meant to be exposed to large amounts of refined foods and sugar, but instead was designed to digest food in such a way that it maximized the sugar that was naturally part of the food itself (and as it digested and released the natural sugars, it got a host of other healthy, beneficial nutrients as well). So the first thing to understand is that sugar in nature is not abundant and always comes as part of a whole-food with many other necessary macro and micro nutrients alongside it.

The second thing to understand is that when you're stressed your body will crave sugar. In terms of survival, when we're stressed, our bodies need a way to access fast burning fuel so it can hit the jets and deal with a true emergency. Since refined sugar wasn't found readily in our environment, our bodies needed a system to hold onto sugar and have it available for quick retrieval. So part of our design is a system of temporary reserves. When you consume carbohydrates, sugar molecules are stored first in a temporary holding situation, so the body always has some reserves ready to release into the blood quickly if it needs it. As you eat more food and new sugar molecules get released in the blood the temporary holding reserve gets stored as longer term reserves in the form of fat, and the new sugar gets moved into the temporary holding reserve. It's an elegant system that served us for many thousands of years. But here's where it gets sticky. Stress is a signal to our bodies that we need to be on high alert and release the quick burning fuel. Stress needs sugar because it doesn't take much energy to process and metabolize, it supplies us with a jolt of energy. It's also the only fuel our brains use to function, so when we're in a threatening situation, we have to keep our brains working well. Stress and sugar are biochemically deeply connected and have been for our whole human existence.

Now, though, we've created a Sahara desert around us in terms of modern food production, with tons of heat in the form of readily available sugary junk food. When we feel stressed, instead of our bodies using the sugar in our temporary reserves, we just reach for the closest sugar fix. We bypass one of our most brilliant designs because we have refined sugar (once rare, now ubiquitous) at such abundant supply. Our bodies were simply not designed to handle chronic stress or chronic digestion of sugar.

## It's Not More Information You Need

So here's the thing—you know that sugar isn't good for you. You know sugar makes you feel stressed, anxious, spacey and gain weight. It isn't for lack of information about food that we have such a conflicted relationship with how to feed ourselves well. The whole time my own health and well being were being drained from the core, I was actually training to become a holistic health coach. Here I was, with a degree in nutrition and biochemistry, a Master's in public health, actively training to become certified in health coaching, and I could barely get through the day without bursting into tears with an infant in my arms, a toddler tugging at my pant leg, and reaching for the coffee pot to refuel.

We don't need more information about food. We need to rewire how we use food in our lives. We need to learn the skill of using food to nourish, cleanse, heal, and rebuild rather than using food to numb out, pacify, or manage difficult feelings. This core essential of a Nourished Body is not about fine tuning your optimal diet. It's not about maximizing your metabolism or fitting into a certain sized pair of jeans. Nor is it about finding the super food extract that will smooth your cellulite. It's about how to protect our deepest wellbeing by the right care of the bodies we are in. From this bedrock, we can fine-tune how we feed ourselves to best fit the bodies we live in, but if we don't take care of the psychology around how we use food in our life, we get tossed into an emotionally tug of war with using food to force our bodies into shape instead of using it to nurture our body.

George MacDonald has written, "You are a soul. You have a body."[5] That's the premise I began to take when I finally established the deep roots of a Nourished Body in my life. I'd consider how I could honor my spirit through how I honored my body. And a crucial part of that was how I fed my body. How you feed yourself is a critical part of replenishing yourself from the inside out. You simply can't experience a vibrant, energized, and calm life living off of Diet Coke and cheese doodles. Every thought, feeling, emotion, reaction, cell, tissue, system, and hormone that is part of your body has a biophysical counterpart—and that biophysical counterpart gets built based on the raw materials you provide your body through the food you eat. My friend and colleague, Dr. Sara Gottfried, author of The Hormone Cure says it this way, "Start with the biology." Before you try to find blame with all your own shortcomings around why you are feeling the way you feel, before you shift into guilt, blame and shame, start with the basic biology of your body—are you giving yourself the raw materials to be well? It's that simple … and that complex. So let's unpack this a little more.

## Food Belongs in Your Body, Not in Your Head

Most of my life I've been trained to think about food, understand it, calculate it, categorize it and keep it in my head space. Things began to change radically when I started listening to my body instead of my head about what foods would best serve, cleanse, and nourish me. But here's what you need to know about this process. When I began to listen to what my body was telling me I needed more of, it didn't necessarily say, "You need kale." But it would say things like, "You feel heavy. You feel congested. You feel weak. You feel tired." Sometimes I could hear distinct cravings like "I want sweet" or "I want salty and crunchy." After a time I saw patterns. Cravings like "I want sweet" were almost always connected to "I'm crazy stressed out right now" or "I'm bored to tears right now."

Let me give you one small example from my life. In a fourteen month span of time, I had sold my home, moved into a rental home for a year, and bought, renovated, and moved into our new home. I was six months pregnant with Brian, our youngest, when we finally settled into our new home. Jackson was just over three years old and Madelyn was sixteen months old. To say that I headed into that winter exhausted is an understatement.

When I was about seven months pregnant I began to have intense cravings for fast food—in particular McDonald's hamburgers. At first I tried to just ignore it. Fast food wasn't part of our lives. At that point, I don't think I could have remembered the last time I drove through a McDonald's. I figured that maybe I was craving red meat, which kind of made sense to me—we were in the winter months, I was very pregnant and while we eat some red meat, it isn't a large part of our diet. So I went out and bought some stew meat and some ground meat as well, and rotated a couple more red meat dishes into our meal plan. But the cravings would not let up. In fact, oddly, when the stew was ready, my stomach turned, I wasn't interested in the meat at all. But still, the strong cravings for drive-through hamburgers continued.

Well, it didn't take long before I went and ordered my hamburgers from McDonald's and ate them as I drove home with two little people in the backseats and one settled nicely on my bladder. As I was eating my burger and fries, I kept wondering, what is this all about, really? Why out of nowhere was I getting these strong cravings. And then a thought hit me like a tsunami wave. The flood gates opened and I found myself stopped at the side of the road on a back street crying my eyes out. It had nothing to do with nutrition at all. I just wanted someone to prepare a meal for me. I was so exhausted, to the bone tired, and had been running full steam on fumes for so long. I was hugely pregnant, with two toddlers, having just made another full house move. It was winter and cold and bleak. And I was just craving someone to make me dinner right now in life. That was it. That's why I wanted that blasted hamburger from McDonald's so badly.

It was a huge lesson for me about cravings and how interconnected we are. And it was a huge lesson for me about how far we'll let ourselves go without checking in and taking care of ourselves along the way. While this example isn't about sugar, it's about how your true cravings will surface if you start looking for them. So let's start by looking at a handful of popular reasons we have sugar cravings so you can begin your detective work.

# 3 Popular (Biological) Reasons to Crave Sugar

We all have our own unique craving fingerprint around why, when and what foods we crave. Understanding what personally triggers you to crave highly processed, sugary foods is an important first step toward dismantling the habit of having these foods as mainstays in your diet. When you can recognize your personal patterns you can begin to pause before reaching for something sugary and consider different ways to fill the underlying need that's present. While we know there are also many emotional reasons we reach for sugar, let's begin exploring some biological reasons. Here are three common physiological reasons women tend to reach for the sweet stuff.

## 1. It makes us feel good.

We crave sugar when we want our moods lifted. In our brains, there are chemicals called neurotransmitters which correlate to our emotions and moods. Carbohydrate-rich foods increase the concentrations of certain neurotransmitters like serotonin, endorphins, and dopamine. Refined sugar is a fast-acting carbohydrate and initially increases the production of these chemicals in our brains. Serotonin brings on feelings of calm, happiness, wellbeing, and satisfaction. Low levels of serotonin are linked with depression and increased appetite. Endorphins are very powerful opiates that produce intense pleasurable feelings. Chocolate is a food that directly increases the level of endorphins we produce. The problem is that the sugar highs are rapidly followed by sugar lows ... the surge in good feeling chemicals is followed by a drop off and our moods plummet. If you find you reach for sugar in order to lift your mood, to start consider bringing in more foods with complex carbohydrates like whole grains, beans, or vegetables.

## 2. We need more energy.

We crave sugar when we're tired. Refined sugar is fast and furious energy, but it leads quickly to the spike/crash cycle. When we binge on sugar, biochemically we burn all that sugar quickly and it leaves our bodies depleted to continue through the day. Our energy needs demand more fuel, so we reach for the next high-sugar meal—keeping us in this cycle of high sugar, spike of energy, fast crash … until the spike of energy just doesn't happen anymore and we bottom out because our bodies simply can't sustain us on empty nutrients all day long. If you need more energy increase the protein and healthy fat in your meals, especially in your breakfast and see if you feel a difference.

## 3. Our body is hungry for nutrients.

We crave sugar because our bodies assume all food comes with nutrients, but refined sugar is devoid of any nutrients. Our bodies need nutrients to complete the digestion process. In order for sugar to be processed, it must actually grab vitamins and minerals from your body's stores to complete its digestion. So sugar robs us of nutrients every time we eat it. This leaves us with an unsatisfied feeling and a need to replace the drained nutrient reserve. We become hungry and crave more food. If we get into the habit of eating overly processed, sugar-rich foods throughout the day, this hunger/nutrient starved cycle continues and we never feel satisfied. If you're starving your body with a diet devoid of nutrients, make the shift into a whole-foods diet, by bringing in calming and building foods like we'll explore next.

Start with biology for a bit as you begin to explore your own sugar craving fingerprint. When you recognize an underlying reason you're reaching for sugar, that's when you can begin to replace a calming food for your typical standby sweet. So let's begin our discussion around what calming foods are and how we can bring them into our diets.

# Calming foods

Now I know you're probably bracing yourself for a complicated dissertation on another theory of how to eat well. We've been raised by the diet industry convincing us that to eat the perfect diet we need to understand and adhere to a complex set of rules about good and bad foods and an equally complex set of rules around how to prepare and eat them. The problem is we've taken one of the most elemental, basic functions of human survival and created such confusion around it, no one feels confident anymore on how to make good choices for themselves and their families. Our first goal, then, is to bring back simple, common sense clarity around food choices.

Calming foods are, in the broadest sense, foods fit for human consumption. Whole, real foods are all potential calming foods. Our bodies recognize them and know how to process, digest and metabolize them. We're starting at the most basic definition, calming foods are whole foods—plants, fruits, seeds and nuts (naturally grown on the earth or in the sea), animals and fish (raised or living in natural settings), and animal products (prepared in traditional ways).

Now I know immediately some of you are raising an eyebrow, questioning whether this particular food group or that should be considered calming. Isn't red meat inflammatory? What about dairy? Can't potatoes raise your blood glucose just like table sugar? And I heard bad things about nightshade vegetables? I get it. Not every single whole food is going to work for you or your body. And not every single whole food is restorative and healthy in abundant amounts. But when you speak about human nutrition, it's important not to immediately start to box everyone in the world into a particular nutritional theory right from the start—pinning some foods as poison, some as tonic. The art comes in understanding how to use the large range of potentially calming, healthy foods to actually respond and create health in your own unique body.

Under the large scope of calming foods falls the full range of vegetables, sea vegetables, fruits, grains, nuts, seeds, legumes, meats, fish, eggs, and dairy. I know at first this seems a little too simplistic, right? That's the secret, Lisa … eat "real" food? Here are a couple thoughts on that. First off, it's actually hard to observe someone who's eating a primarily whole-foods diet who's also struggling with the effects of chronic depletion. Most often, like the plastic balls in the pool example, shifting your diet to whole, real foods impacts your emotional wellbeing radically. From that point, it's a fantastic idea to fine-tune and optimize your diet based on how your body best responds to different foods, but the first step is always to bring the majority of your diet under the umbrella of whole-foods. Secondly, it doesn't feel simplistic to the person addicted to a high sugar, process-laden diet to shift to a real foods diet. While it may be simple in concept, in our current culture it requires many rewritten habits around food to put healthy eating back into practice again.

Finally, just because a food is under the calming foods umbrella doesn't mean every body works well with every kind of food. We know that isn't true. You are as bio-unique as I am and part of your journey to having a thriving relationship with food is to take the time to explore what works best for you, how much and when. I can assure you that as you dial down the noise of sugar and processed foods in your diet, you will "hear" how your body responds to other foods much more clearly.

So the first step is to move your diet away from chemicalized, sugary, highly processed foods and toward consuming more calming foods—real, whole, true—nutrient dense foods. The mainstays of your diet should be from within this large whole foods umbrella. The next level of nuance we'll add is to explore two more categories of calming foods: the cleansing foods and the building foods. Once you calm your system and the inner noise of an overly processed diet, with whole-foods you can do the work of exploring what types of calming foods work best for what you most need at the moment.

## Cleansing and Building Types of Calming Foods

Within the larger range of calming foods, some will have more of a cleansing quality and some will have more of a building quality. In different traditions, these distinctions sometimes are explained as yin and yang or expansive and contractive. I enjoy using the terms cleansing and building because they related well to the two extremes I often felt when I was imbalanced. I often either felt physically heavy and mentally stuck, or I felt physically weak and mentally spacey. As you get better at checking in with yourself and asking, "What do I need right now?" you'll start to hear a distinction between when you feel sluggish versus when you feel frail. This is a great first step as you learn how to understand food's intrinsic qualities. And we intuitively use food to help us recalibrate all the time. When we're in the middle of a hot, sticky summer, our bodies crave fresh fruits, the juicier the better. The natural sugars in these fruits actually have a cooling characteristic and work well to hydrate and cool our bodies. In the winter months, we gravitate toward heavier foods that are cooked and stewed to provide the antidote for the cold winter temperature for our bodies. This new way of relating to food is as natural and intuitive as you can get, we've just gotten disconnected from our intuitive wisdom.

The final thing to note is that we all need both cleansing and building foods in our diets. It's not a black or white discussion around which foods are cleansers and which are builders. You'll see some types of foods are both. It's simply a subtle way to explore the art of nourishing yourself with whole foods which are meant to help keep our bodies in deeper harmony by responding to our own inner needs, cycles, and seasons we find ourselves in.

## The Cleansers

The cleansers are those foods that help your body remove excess weight and excess mucus or congestion. The cleansers also can help your mind get unstuck when it feels slow and full of cobwebs. In general, foods that are naturally high in fiber and detoxifying properties have cleansing properties, which includes whole-foods like vegetables (especially leafy ones), fruits (especially berries, apples and pears), legumes, seeds, whole grains, algae, and seaweed. Here's a select list of some power house cleansers within the larger umbrella of cleansing foods.

## The Super Cleansers

### *The Green Machines*

- *Dark leafy greens like kale, collard greens, Swiss chard, dandelion greens, and beet greens.*
- *Salad greens like spinach, arugula, watercress, and romaine.*

### *The Sulphurs*

- *Onion, garlic, leeks and chives*

### *Grains and Seeds*

- *Brown Rice*
- *Quinoa*
- *Hemp seeds*
- *Chia Seeds*
- *Pumpkin Seeds*

## Algae

- *Blue-Green algae*
- *Chlorella*
- *Spirulina*

## Seaweed

- *Kombu*
- *Seaweed flakes*
- *Nori*
- *Wakame*

## Spices

- *Ginger*
- *Cayenne*
- *Mustard*
- *Cinnamon*
- *Turmeric*
- *Rosemary*

## Teas

- *Milk Thistle*
- *Dandelion Root*

# The Builders

The builders are excellent to grab when you're feeling weak, depleted, and nutrient starved. They're also helpful when stress is causing you to shift into escape mode and your mind feels spacey and scattered. Builders will help ground you. The whole foods which have a stronger building quality are healthy proteins, healthy fats, dark leafy greens, deeply colored vegetables, natural sources of probiotics, algae, and seaweeds.

# The Super Builders

### *The Green Machines*

- *Dark leafy greens like kale, collard greens, Swiss chard, dandelion greens, and beet greens.*

### *Deep Colored Veggies*

- *Red and purple berries, yams and sweet potatoes, pomegranates, purple grapes, cherries*

### *Healthy Protein*

- *Wild caught and mercury/toxin free fish*
- *Pastured and naturally raised meat and dairy*
- *Organic, free roaming eggs*
- *Broth from the bones of pastured and naturally raised meat*

### *Natural Sources of Probiotics*

- *Plain organic yogurt*
- *Organic kefir*
- *Cultured Vegetables*
- *Miso Soup*
- *Tempeh*
- *Kimchi*
- *Kombucha Tea*

## Omega 3 Fats

- *Wild fatty fish like salmon, tuna, sardines or mackerel*
- *Walnuts*
- *Ground flax seeds*
- *Chia seeds*

## Other Healthy Fats

- *Coconut Oil*
- *Avocado*

## Algae

- *Blue-Green algae*
- *Chlorella*
- *Spirulina*

## Seaweed

- *Kombu*
- *Seaweed flakes*
- *Nori*
- *Wakame*

## Tea

- *Nettles*

These lists are not here to encourage you to become restrictive with your diet and only include these foods in your diet. The idea is to begin to learn simple ways to make food choices reflect what you need most. Here are a few examples on how you can use food in this way.

- You're coming home from a long day of work in the middle of winter. Your mood feels heavy, you've dealt with excess bloating all week, and you're just in a slump. You pause and ask, what would make me feel better right now? You take a quick assessment and decide to lean into some cleansing foods. Because it's winter, you'll cook them—so you make a quick sauté of garlic and greens to have with your supper.

- You just spent a weekend in celebration mode and are feeling the effects of all the sugary foods you ate. Your body is in need of nutrient replenishment. Your mind is feeling spacey and frazzled. So you choose to have an egg and spinach omelet for breakfast and prepare a healthy trail mix with nuts and seeds for your mind-morning snack to start the day.

- You've had a rough couple of weeks (or months) of high stress and it's beginning to catch up with you. Your body feels jittery and anxious. Your mind is jumbled and stuck in negative spirals. You pay attention to the signs of adrenal fatigue and seek to nourish yourself with foods that deliver a mineral-packed punch. As you cook your pot of rice you drop in a few strips of Kombu seaweed. You make a big pot of simple, nourishing soup by sautéing garlic, seaweed flakes and mushrooms in organic butter, tossing in chopped up kale and adding natural chicken broth to a simmer. You'll enjoy a bowl of this soup once or twice a day for the week.

These are uncomplicated, small ways to align the way you nourish yourself with the process of actually paying attention to yourself and what your needs are right now—while tapping into the power and wisdom of whole foods. I know that major changes to our diet don't happen overnight or often after reading a chapter in a book. That's why I began my wellness work with mothers all over the world by teaching courses that explored these principles in a step by step journey over time. If you'd like to learn more about my courses, I've included more information about them in the appendix. And if eating for a vibrant life is something you're particularly interested in, I encourage you to learn more about my Designed for Wellness course.

# Respond to Your Inner Needs

Anytime we take on something like changing the way we feed ourselves, it's useful to have simple guidelines to follow as we re-establish new habits in our life. It gives us a starting place and, perhaps even more importantly, a place to return to when we fall back into old patterns and need to course correct. Here are four simple steps I come back to every time I find myself needing to correct how I'm using food in my life.

## 1. Pause and Check-In

Get used to pausing and checking in. This is simply the art of curiously asking yourself what is happening in your body and mind. It is taking a moment before putting something in your mouth to be intentional about it. It's recognizing an opportunity to nourish and care for yourself through how you feed yourself. At first you may not have a large vocabulary around describing how you are feeling. That's okay. Start with whatever descriptions come to mind. Does your body feel heavy and sluggish? Are you experiencing tightness, tension or anxiety? Is your mind wandering and spacey? Are your thoughts slow and unfocused? Just this simple step of taking note of how you are feeling is an act of care and attention to your wellbeing.

One of the best places to begin is to create this pause by reaching first for water before you eat. You can even personalize this step as well. My starting point was from a place of feeling very weak, depleted, and easily chilled. So I catered how I hydrated myself to reflect my need for warmer nourishment. I began by sipping hot water and lemon throughout my day. Sometimes I would add a touch of honey and a spoonful of Braggs apple vinegar. Sometimes when the lemons ran out, I'd just sip plain hot water. But the warmth and the moisture from the steam warmed me. Just holding a warm cup in the mornings and throughout my day settled me, calmed me, and made me feel wrapped in care. Just a small act, but a small act of care toward myself went a long way from where I was.

## 2. Bring in the Good

The second step I worked on was to bring in calming foods. As I shifted out of the stronghold sugar and caffeine had on my body and mind, I started each day focused on bringing in as many foods as I could that would calm the noise inside and nourish me. I can remember writing out a handful of grounding, healthy foods that I wanted to get in each day. For a while I ate them right alongside the crap. I had my eggs and sautéed greens along with three cups of coffee and a mid morning handful of Honey Nut Cheerios. But I ate my eggs and greens so I felt great about myself. All through my day I singularly focused on what I was going to bring in and allowed myself to eat anything else that I wanted—I just wouldn't replace the good stuff with the crap. I didn't worry too much about eating them side by side. This strategy disarmed my addictions faster than anything I'd tried before. Because it steadied and nourished my body to get calming foods in, I was so much more equipped to break from the sugar addiction and move fully into a nourishing diet.

## 3. Slow Down

My third step was to become more mindful of how I was eating. As a mom of little ones, there were days I consumed every bite of food standing up or running out the door. I knew I wanted to reverse this pattern that kept me connecting food with high stress, so I would commit at least one meal a day where I sat down and ate a meal without rushing. Many times I'd light a candle, eat slowly and enjoy feeding my body good and wholesome food. One of my tricks was to make a deal with myself that whenever I craved something with high sugar, I could have it as long as I sat down and ate it slowly, enjoying every bite.

## 4. Refine and Align

Align your food choices with what your body, mood, and mind truly need. This is the step where I asked myself throughout the day how I was feeling and what I needed most. I learned more about the inner qualities of foods and saw the power of using food choices to balance, heal, and harmonize on the most fundamental level. This is part of the work I do with women in my course, Designed for Wellness. Working week by week and learning about how different foods impact your wellbeing and being able to make intuitive wise choices about what to eat is incredibly exciting and freeing for many women who've been stuck in patterns of struggle and battle with food for much of their lives.

## Keep Food as a Tool

I know many "health nuts" that are far from healthy. I know people who eat cleaner diets than I can even conceive of eating, walking around without a glimpse of joy, sometimes thin to the point of frail bodies, or with a constant sense of anxiety and insecurity around what they feed themselves. This is not health or vitality. This is not using your prosperity of health to bless your own life and overflow into goodness for others. As soon as a tool (in this case healthy food) becomes the end goal, it is corrupted and corrupts. As soon as you no longer use food to keep yourself well and vital, but instead generate an obsession around consuming healthy food, you have shifted from using food as a tool into using it as a weapon.

One way food's sold to us as a weapon is through the "easy tweak." Blasted from commercials and plastered on magazine covers, we are constantly promised that lure of easy, quick results with just one little magic bullet addition to our diet. We hear about a little-heard-of vitamin that immediately corrects raging moods. Or a secret super food that clears out cellulite. The promise of the easy tweak is really the myth of the easy tweak. Here's why. Tweaks only produce real change when our foundations are strong and well established. A can of paint really can do wonders for a room—but that assumes the walls aren't falling down. I think it's in our nature to want major change without majorly changing. I get it. And I also know that to try majorly changing a life that already feels tapped to the brim seems overwhelming. The difference between an easy tweak that falls short of real change and small shifts that produce huge results is where the changes are directed. Direct your small steps toward building up your foundations first and you will see massive success.

In this chapter we explored some powerful ways to replenish the core essential of a Nourished Body by fixing the cracks in the foundation first. Remember that every time you make a choice to more deeply care for yourself, you are turning on a hose. All those trickles add up and before you know it you're feeling lighter and more buoyant. In this way, food is one of the many tools you're gathering in your satchel for the journey—and when you use the tool of nourishing food be mindful to hold it well so it heals, calms, and nurtures you in all ways. Here is a quick overview of the strategies we explored around the Nourished Body core essential.

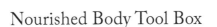

## Nourished Body Tool Box

- *Explore your personal cravings fingerprint*
- *Move your diet first under the whole foods umbrella*
- *Slow down – Begin to eat slowly and while sitting*
- *Begin asking yourself, "How am I feeling?" and "What would make my body feel best right now?"*
- *Refine your food choices within the cleansing and building categories*
- *Keep food as a tool for your wellbeing*

# Chapter 5
# Restorative Rest

My husband, Mike, works as a police officer on the night shift. One night, after a particularly difficult day, he came through the door at 3:00 am and found me zoned out in front of the computer at the kitchen table. I'd been woken up a couple hours earlier by my daughter needing to nurse. When I woke, I found myself hanging off my son's toddler bed, where I'd crashed out after trying to get him to sleep earlier in the night. After nursing Madelyn and putting her back down, I worried I would just end up tossing and turning for hours back in my own bed—sleep deprivation had a way of turning into insomnia for me in the middle of the night. So I hopped on the computer to get lost in some artificially-lit surfing for a while.

When Mike found me, he put his arms around me and held me for a while. Then he turned me toward him and said, "Hon, you have to start taking advantage of every hour you can rest. You can't control all your broken sleep, but you have control over this." It must have been that every word he spoke was dripping with genuine concern and compassion that I didn't stiffen and lash back at him, quipping something sarcastic and defensive. This time something in me softened. Something shifted and I knew he was right.

In this core essential of Restorative Rest, we'll explore rest for your body. So often, when we find ourselves in emotionally and mentally dry and exhausted places, we believe that only a major change will ever bring about real relief. During a MAPP (Motherhood, Ambition, Passion and Purpose) Gathering interview I conducted with best-selling author and teacher, Jennifer Louden, she shared that, "when you feel a lack of passion or you have this lost feeling or you feel like running away … go back and ask, 'How am I doing with my minimum requirements of self-care?' because sometimes it's simply the fact you haven't had a good night's sleep in a year."[6] Until I came to the honest place that I was squandering the little I could do for myself in this core area of wellbeing, things never got better. I believe that self care is truly an act of self stewardship. Ultimately, it's choosing to care for the gift of yourself and your own health. It's an act of generosity rather than greed. And stewardship always begins with taking good care of the little you have in order to gain more of what you truly want. If there's one core essential moms feel they have least control over, it's often the core essential of Restorative Rest … and that's exactly why giving ourselves even a little care in this area produces the greatest amount of positive impact.

## Rest for Your Body

In his fantastic book, Brain Rules, developmental molecular biologist, John Medina, tells the story of seventeen year old high school student, Randy Gardner's, high school science-fair project that landed him in the Guinness Book of World Records.[7] Gardner decided to forgo any sleep for eleven straight days to observe what happens during acute sleep deprivation. As I read the impact of this study on Randy's mind and body, I began to realize how serious the lack of sleep is to our basic functioning. Very quickly, Randy began to feel irritable, forgetful, and nauseous ... not to mention tired. Five days in, the impacts on his cognition resembled Alzheimer's disease. He was also actively hallucinating and severely disoriented. By the end of his project his fingers were trembling and his speech slurred. I believe this is more than an interesting anecdote. How many times have you gone through your day with excessive irritation, forgetfulness and nausea and never considered it was simply a symptom of a poor night's sleep? Could improving your rest (even by small increments) really impact your wellbeing in such powerful ways? The answer is yes. The core essential of Restorative Rest is a critical way we can trickle true replenishment into our lives.

It would've been easy for me to feel my hands were tied in this area— wait, let me rewrite that. It was easy to feel my hands were tied around rest and sleep given the season of life I was in with such little children—and so, consequently, I released any personal responsibility to do the little I could to support myself in this area.   The old patterns of perfectionism began surfacing in my life and because I couldn't conceive of getting the kind of rest that I wanted, I gave up on trying to get better rest. If you struggle with perfectionism like I do, as soon as you notice you've been giving up on something important because you can't do it perfectly, try to reframe the situation and ask yourself, "What would my personal best be right now in this situation or about this area of my life?" When your goal is your personal best, you're freed up to consider what author of the blog Simple Mom, Tsh Oxenreider calls "partial solutions."[8] Solutions that solve at least a little of the problem and move you a little closer to the place you want to be, even if your ideal or perfect solution can't be met.

Holding out for the opportunity to get perfect rest ended up only getting me further and further into dark and desperate days. The evening my husband named the truth of the situation, and I was ready to receive it, I saw so clearly that it may not be perfect, but I could do a whole lot more than I was doing to care for myself in this area—I was certainly not going for my personal best.

So I began to look at my own contribution to the sleep deprivation I was feeling. I explored if there may be any little way I could ease the intensity I was feeling. And that was a saving grace moment for me. What I found is your sleep doesn't have to be perfect for you to feel huge improvement in regeneration … indeed small efforts to improve the true rest you offer your body and mind will give back in spades.

## Forming the Habit of Poor Sleep

Here's one of the other problems with this all or nothing attitude around sleep and rest that can get established early on: As a new mom, it's a human life that's keeping you from having the sleep your body needs to function optimally. But left unchecked, we can use this as a crutch and a slippery slope. Because we're already sleep deprived, we can let down our guard and allow all sorts of trespasses into our lives that continue to suck the life out of us.

So we fall into a pattern of sleep deprivation. And then years after the kids are sleeping through the night, we're still tossing and turning, waking in the middle of the night and can't get back to sleep, staying up way too late in front of brightly lit screens, or acting like productivity machines running ourselves on high speed until the moment we hit the bed. When you take back the reigns in this area of your life—regardless of what season you find yourself in—you rewrite the capacity to experience rest and renewal which can serve you for many years in the future. A chronically sleep deprived momma simply can't function anywhere close to how she is meant to. You've heard the adage, small hinges swing big doors. The small hinges we'll talk about may at first seem like a drop in the ocean against the level of exhaustion you feel, but trust this process. Offer up the little you have and you'll be blown away by how much you receive in return.

## Bed Time Routines

As parents we're well versed with the need for bed time routines for our children. We see in real time that asking our kids to go to bed right after they've been highly stimulated is a losing proposal. Intuitively (and experientially) we understand going to sleep is not like flipping a switch. It helps to have external cues that signal a slowing down to your system, a settling in, a retreating from the day's activities and a preparation for deep rest. In fact this is exactly how it happens biochemically. Melatonin, which is the primary hormone responsible for your ability to shut off wakefulness and enter into restorative sleep should slowly increase beginning at the hours around sunset, allowing you to enter a restful sleep at bedtime, which is, ideally, before 11:00 pm. There tends to be a tipping point for each of us when we're finally able to shift into sleep during the evening hours and the production of melatonin is a big factor in this. Melatonin is highly responsive to environmental triggers. So whereas our bodies used to respond to the cycles of natural sunlight, artificial light has influenced our melatonin production and impacted our circadian rhythms. When our circadian rhythms are off we can either have a hard time falling to sleep, wake up in the middle of the night to insomnia, or feel tired all day even after a full night's sleep.

The good news is that an effective wind down routine can be both enjoyable and compact. It doesn't have to be long, complex, or difficult to put better sleep habits into practice. The hard part, of course, is the commitment to it. The prioritizing of it. Because as moms we have just So. Much. To. Get. Done. Many of us argue the only time we get a foothold on our never ending list of stuff is in the late evening hours. I get that. I had convinced myself I had to do work in the evening hours. I was building a business while raising three little kids, and nights were when I had the time to do my work. And in truth, there were many hours in the evening that did need to be earmarked for work, but once I began to dig a little deeper, there were areas of fat that could be cut. You need an honest assessment of how you're really doing. For a very long time I was functioning under severe sleep deprivation and the quality of everything else was impacted. Giving a little to this core essential area of my wellbeing ended up paying me in spades with increased calm, vitality, focus, and productivity. Sometimes you simply have to stop chopping down the tree and sharpen the blade.

## Sacred Book Ends

I want you to think about your evenings as a sacred bookend to your day. Establishing an evening routine to prepare your body and mind for sleep is a powerful way to bring more restoration and healing into your life. Many women I work with feel at a loss on how to set up an effective evening routine, so here's a simple template to begin with.

Think of your evening routine as taking you over a bridge from where you are at the end of the day to a place where your body and mind are ready to fall into a deeper level of rest. So the first thing to do is consider where you're starting from as you begin to wind down from the day. Most of us are very stimulated and connected to our outer world from the day. After being engaged in the world all day long, the goal of your evening routine is to slowly disengage you from the world and bring you back inward to yourself to ready yourself for deep restorative sleep.

Let's say part of what you need to get done in the evening is work, either business related or home related. It could be anything from computer work, phone calls, household chores or projects. Give yourself time as early in the evening as possible to focus on those things. Create clear boundaries around your work or home time so there's a start and stop time. This also makes your evening work time more efficient—you're more likely to focus in and get the most important things done when you have a clear time limit for your work.

Once your work time is done, move one step inward and do something to calm your physical body. This can be very simple, even the act of washing up, getting into PJs, and moisturizing your face is a way to acknowledge you're readying your body for sleep. Things that soothe your central nervous system like we explored earlier, for example a long warm bath, a hot towel scrub, or a foot massage are simply ways to soothe your body. I love to do a simple self massage, light stretching, or simple yoga postures as well. Another strategy is to turn off or dim the lights around the house during this time. Artificial light disrupts the production of melatonin, so softening the light around you is an excellent part of your evening routine. In fact, this has been extremely helpful as I ready my kids for bed as well. About thirty minutes to an hour before I want them in bed, I'll turn off all screens and dim the lights in the house. We begin to do calmer activities like reading or coloring as we transition into our bedtime routines.

Next in your personal evening routine, go one layer further inward and consider ways to calm and relax your mind. I love to tap into the master calming techniques like we explored with our Calm Mind core essential to establish a deep calm throughout my limbic system. Actions like inspirational reading, meditation, or journaling can also help calm and ready your mind for deep rest. Using essential oils can be particularly powerful to calm and relax your mind. This is an especially important element to include if you find your mind races as soon as you hit the pillow. Allowing space to get your thoughts out of your head and into a journal gives them a place to go and creates more calm and peace in your mind.

Finally end with nurturing your spirit. I love including something right before bed that aligns with my spirit and symbolizes what I want to bring more of into my life. Gratitude journaling is fantastic at the end of the day. Recently I've discovered an app for my phone, Omvana, which allows you to record your own voice with soothing music in the background.[9] So I recorded prayers, Scripture, and inspiring words to listen to right before I drift to sleep.

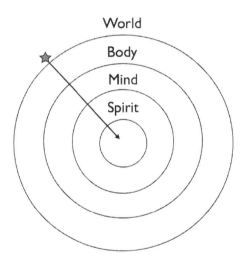

# The Evening Routine Template

Here's what the above evening routine might look like.

8:00 pm: Respond to work emails.

8:30 pm: Put in a load of laundry, clean up the kitchen.

9:00 pm: Dim the lights around the house. PJs, wash face

and brush teeth (if you haven't done this when your kids were doing it!). Give yourself a 5 minute foot rub with warm coconut oil. Do a few simple stretches.

9:25 pm: Get out your journal and spend some time writing. End with a small list of gratitudes from the day.

9:45 pm: In bed, grab some light reading—maybe an inspirational book or scripture.

10:00 pm: Lights off and slip off to sleep.

This is just a simple template to work through as you consider how to craft a meaningful bedtime routine that results in deeper, more restorative rest. This doesn't have to take a long time. I can do a couple of these things even in twenty-thirty minutes. I prefer giving myself a full hour but it isn't necessary. It's the consistency, the predictability, and the new habit of prioritizing the care of yourself at the closing of your day. The symbol of saying your days are important and the closing of a day is something to be marked intentionally with loving care. On a biochemical level, giving yourself a sacred book end of an evening routine resets your circadian rhythm by allowing your melatonin production to rise in the evening. Melatonin is a critical hormone not only important for getting sleep, but also in your ability to stay asleep throughout the night. Sometimes we don't think we have problems sleeping because we hit the bed and fall immediately to sleep, but we wake in the middle of the night and have a hard time returning to sleep, or we wake after a night's sleep and feel un-refreshed and tired every morning. How you prepare yourself for sleep makes a huge difference in these cases.

## When You Go to Sleep Matters

Before the advent of artificial light, our sleep patterns were firmly tethered to the natural cycle of daylight. Everyone does have their own sweet spot of time to sleep and wake. Sleep researchers predict about thirty percent of the population are on the extremes—either waking very early (with early bedtimes) or waking late (with late bedtimes). The rest of us likely do best in the 10:00 pm bed-time and 6:00 am wake-time range. There's a whole science around finding your sleep cycles and aligning your times of sleep and times of wake to coordinate with them. But I'm a firm believer of keeping first steps simple. If you're chronically under-rested and are going to bed later than 11:00 pm most evenings, a great first step is to move your bedtime back as much as possible. You can even do this in small increments. If you go to sleep ten minutes earlier every night, it takes less than a week to shift a whole hour. In fact, consider a simple experiment for one week where you do just that. Each night aim to be in bed completely ready for sleep ten minutes earlier than you were the night before. Give yourself one-two full weeks for this experiment so you can explore a range of bedtimes and waking times. Note each morning how you feel upon waking. Note also the energy you feel throughout the day and see if you can pinpoint a sleep time that works best for you.

## When Kids Do It, You Do It.

Bedtimes in our home can feel like an ever-changing swirl of hoops we need to jump through just to get our kids settled, watch their eyes finally close and call it a day. For the longest time I would shuffle my three little ones through the drill: pajamas on, brush teeth, wipe down face or take a bath, read books, sip of water, then the ever-changing tuck in process which ranged from sitting in chairs outside their room, sitting in lotus position next to their beds (my attempt at multi-tasking meditation, it doesn't work, by the way), sleeping with them, rubbing backs, prayers, and escorting escapees back into their beds over and over again.

Finally, once they were asleep, I'd still be in my day clothes (which, six times out of seven, would now double as my PJs), and all too often I'd climb into my own bed without so much as brushing my teeth or washing my face. If I took out my contacts I'd call it a good night. I don't know why it took me so long to figure out one of the simplest strategies of all—get yourself ready for bed while you're getting the kids ready for bed. This one little shift started a huge change in my own evening experience. Now when the kids get in PJs, I do too. Now when the kids brush their teeth, I do too. Now when they take a bath, I wash my face, I moisturize, I take a hot towel and essential oils and give my neck and shoulders a nice rub down. Now before I shuffle them toward their rooms, I take my contacts out and put on my glasses. Even if I find myself at midnight hanging off a toddler bed with drool plastered on my cheek, at least my mouth feels fresh, my face feels clean, and after I make it back to my own room, I'm climbing under my own sheet with PJs on. This is my non-negotiable now for a bedtime routine. For a while this was all I could do … heck, this was amazing—this was a huge step in my own self care. We have to start where we are and build from there. Wherever you are, don't fight it, just start with the first step in front of you.

## Rest During the Day

Let's talk about rest during the day. Ok I can just feel it; I can feel your eyes roll. I get how insane this sounds at first, it almost sounds like a joke to tell moms to rest during the day. This is all the more why we have to talk about it. Why do we expect our bodies to be run like machines? Why do we expect that we can go non-stop all day long and have any honest connections to the natural rhythms and cycles of our lives? And why do we feel so guilty when we slow down?

# How to Slow Down

I want you to think about when you naturally feel exhausted during the day. Where are your slumps? Chances are they'll be in one of two places. Either they're during times when you have a moment to slow down and you'll feel like you just bottomed out. Like you spent the whole day carrying the weight of the world on your shoulders and now that there's not an immediate fire to put out, you collapse. Or it can happen right in the middle of the most intense parts of your day. During the morning rush when you're still gulping coffee and trying to shake yourself out of sleep. Or maybe those after-school-into-dinner hours when everyone is in mental meltdown mode and life really picks up with practices, meals, and homework. In each of these scenarios, when we feel excessive exhaustion surface, it's a sign we're burning out our adrenals. Over time, our adrenal glands simply can't keep up and even when we need them most, they don't fire up— making high-stress times even more intense and unbearable.

We're not meant to race with our foot on the gas pedal all day long, yet we've completely lost this wisdom in our current culture. Even short breaks and small doses of limbic calming throughout the day make huge differences in our overall vitality. What if you took one day and wrote out an hour-by-hour schedule from waking to sleeping? Now, before you fill in your day, first write in a handful of times when you will commit to taking a small break to mindfully relax, retreat and fill the well in some meaningful way. Perhaps it's sitting on the couch, eyes closed, feet up, and deeply breathing for five minutes. Maybe it's getting on the ground and stretching or inverting your legs up the wall in a calming yoga pose for three minutes. What if you penciled in a ten minute walk around the block before the kids got home from school? Think about writing in your times of restoration first and then fitting in all that must be done in a day around them. For even one day, give it a shot and see what difference you experience.

One suggestion I give to moms who feel they're at a loss for ways to slow down and take time to restore in the gaps of their day is to write out a "Mini-Renewal" list on a piece of paper and keep it on the fridge. I generally say have two columns. One column should be things that can be done in ten minutes or under, the other column is for things that can be done in thirty minutes or under. Keep a growing list of small tools and strategies you're learning about that can become little moments of replenishment throughout your day. Have it posted where you won't forget it and when a gap opens in your day, you can look to the list for ideas and inspiration.

## Honoring the Ebb and Flow

On the most primary, physical level the core essential of Restorative Rest expresses itself as a need for physical rest through proper, restorative sleep. But this core essential has deep layers that reflect the kind of rest your mind, mood and spirit also need to experience. In essence it also reflects the natural need for our lives to have a healthy ebb and a healthy flow. Our times of rest and retreat are like our in-breath. It's reflected in the wisdom of the seasons to have a winter, in the moon to wane in a dark sky, in the seed to take it's time deep in the earth before it sprouts. It's written in the wisdom of our bodies as our eggs drop inward wrapped in the swell of our uterus before releasing outward in our monthly hormonal cycles.

We live in a culture that reveres the out-breath, so it takes a conscious decision to shift the rhythm of your life to allow for both the in and out-breath to be honored. Thankfully you don't need to have perfect sleep before you can enjoy the benefits of better sleep. You don't need to have a three-day weekend at a resort spa before you can commit time for rest, reflection and receiving in your everyday life. It's the small trickles that fill the pond. Take stock of where you land on the ebb and flow spectrum most of your days. If you tend toward chronic out-breath consider what small shift you can bring in today to balance the scales a little and find the flow and vitality from a well-rounded full breath cycle. Here's a quick summary of the tools we explored to bolster the core essential of Restorative Rest in our lives.

## Restorative Rest Tool Box

- *Drop the perfectionist snare and commit to small shifts in this area*

- *Create a simple evening routine using the*

- *World–Body–Mind–Spirit Model*

- *Explore getting to sleep earlier, preferably before 11:00 pm*

- *Prepare for bedtime with your kids*

- *Allow times of rest and renewal to punctuate your day*

- *Create a "Mini-Renewal" list to have ideas ready for small gaps of downtime in your day*

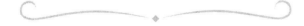

# Chapter 6

# Joyful Movement

Even though I was on the phone, I could feel Tracy hold her breath when I suggested we talk about healthy movement in her life. It was effortless for us to dive into other core essentials during our earlier calls. Tracy was on board with feeding her body vital, life-giving foods. Together, we explored establishing better sleep routines and self reflective practices. But now I felt the layers of resistance come up and bring a lifetime of confusion, frustration, and pain to the surface.

"I'm not an athlete, never have been really, although there have been times I've stuck with a workout plan for a while by forcing myself to. I just don't like exercise. But I'll do it, I know it's important."

As soon as I heard these words I knew the path to freedom for Tracy in this area of her life was completely opposite what she thought she needed to do. What I heard was the good girl who wants to please, who'll force herself and her body to do something because she knows it's good for her. I heard the one who wants to be the good student and not disappoint the coach. So it was a total shock when I suggested we start with her wardrobe. Before we can truly relish the joy of moving our glorious bodies for the sake of joy alone, we have to begin relating to our bodies with authentic love, with authentic appreciation, with authentic delight. From there we can reacquaint ourselves with the sheer brilliance of having bodies that can move and stretch and sweat. But if we get this order wrong, we end up using movement and activity as a weapon against ourselves to whip us into shape, and to force ourselves to be something we're currently not.

It's good to challenge yourself and to increase your body's capacity for cardiovascular stamina and physical strength, but there's a difference when it's sourced from an honest interest and natural ambition to push yourself farther toward growth versus a sense of obligation and drudgery. I'm all for working out and getting in fantastic athletic shape. But I also know our need for simple movement we truly enjoy is at the heart of filling your core essential of Joyful Movement, which we're going to explore more deeply here.

## Listen to What Your Body Wants

My desire for movement has run the gamut from intense training on the asphalt to slow walks in the woods. The hardest part has always been dropping the external definitions of what "in shape" means and listening inward for my body to tell me how it wants to move.

Nine months after I gave birth to my first son I ran a triathlon. It just felt right. I always had a personal goal to complete a triathlon. When my son was six months old, I began thinking about that goal again. It was also at a time in my life when the newness of a baby dissembled any structure there used to be to the rhythms of my days. I couldn't tell you when I'd get to brushing my teeth from one day to the next. Part of what I loved about deciding to do the triathlon was it automatically brought back some structure to my days. It also concretely roped my husband into giving me specific times when I could work out and he would watch Jackson, a respite in my weeks that I desperately needed. My body, mind, and spirit were totally in with this goal and I honestly loved every part of the process from getting started on training to getting across the finish line.

After my second and then my third child, the last thing I cared about was taking on another physical challenge like a triathlon. I wondered if my body was ever going to feel the rush of being strong, lean, and energized again, but it was exhausting just to think of exercise as a priority. Before I could care for my body the way I needed to, I had to reconnect with what I was truly craving in this area of my life. I yearned for dance, for yoga, for walks in the woods, for stretching, for rebounding, for regaining the expression of my femininity through the delightful movement of my body. I wanted to wrap my body with colors and textures that felt beautiful to me. More than ever before, I wanted to feel sensual again in my skin. This time around, the core essential of Joyful Movement took a completely different route. Had I forced myself into a more traditional definition of physical exercise it would've been one dead end after another. Instead I let my heart lead me to how my body wanted to express itself.

Just like with my work with Tracy, sometimes the place to begin is how you're treating your body, right now as it is. That's why we started with wardrobe and how she felt toward her body in the here and now. If you're unsure what your body actually craves, begin with the end in mind. Imagine yourself at your ideal weight and size. Imagine yourself strong and lean, flexible and energized. Imagine how you would treat your body then. What colors will you wear? What style of clothes would you put on every day? Would you moisturize more often after the shower? Would you give your body more exfoliating scrubs? Take more baths? Wear sexier nightgowns? Walk with better posture? When you shift your actions to align with loving your body now, your body can more freely let you know how it wants to feel and how it wants to move. You get a much clearer sense how this core essential wants to be filled and replenished.

What I found along the way is that every time I allowed the core essential of Joyful Movement to come into my life in this delight-led way, more often than not, it naturally led to a higher level of physical activity in my life. And once the internal motivator was ignited, my workouts happened without the mental barriers of resistance and force. So if you're in a place where your needs for Joyful Movement are not being met, let's break it down to three simple principles that shift the perspective around healthy movement and get us moving forward. These simple shifts in perspective will guide us to know exactly how our bodies most want to move: start where you are interested, start where you are, keep it simple.

## Step 1: Start Where You're Interested

I want you to imagine a scenario where no one is looking. Let's say you have a full month on a deserted island. You're completely safe, your needs are provided for, and you get to spend your days doing what you want, simply for yourself. No one is judging, in fact, no one will ever know how you spent your time. You have plenty of rest; you have plenty of time eating healthy, delicious, fresh foods. You have no stressors in your life, no obligations, no deadlines, and no difficult interactions.

Now decide how you want to explore and move through your day. Would you swim, would you take long walks on the shoreline? Would you hike the forested mountains? Would you climb the trees? Would you surf on the waves? Would you scramble on rock faces? Would you dance? Would you stretch? Would you do yoga poses among the wildflowers? Would you retreat into the fully air-conditioned hut and hop on the treadmill or pop in an aerobics workout DVD? Would you bounce on a trampoline or strap roller skates to your feet?

Roll this visioning exercise around in your mind. A fantastic idea to experience this exercise more fully is to begin a vision board and clip out images of movement that feel exciting to you. Don't worry if you feel you can do these things right now … just allow yourself to drawn in what feels good to you. Connect feelings of excitement and desire around healthy movement in your mind. Open to the possibility that you'll soon have a strong, vibrant body that delights in movement. Yes, you need to start where you are and yes, you need to start with the options around you. Maybe you're feeling far from capable of doing what you'd love to be able to do. Maybe you can only stretch your mind in small reaches, and your vision is about sitting on a grassy slope, stretching your legs and taking a long nap. This isn't about anyone else's journey but your own. But the only way to bring healthier, more sustainable movement into your life is when it draws you toward it, not when you have to push yourself into it. And the way to do that is to encourage your mind to grab a hold of the possibility that you'll feel delight when you engage in activity and movement.

In my mind's eye, on that deserted tropical island, I'd climb rocks and swim in the rivers. I'd hike mountain tops and stretch on sandy sun-soaked stretches of shoreline. But as I'm writing this I'm in New Jersey, in the middle of a cold and grey winter. No sign of sun and space and stress-free living in sight. So while my tropical wonderland isn't an option right now, I do know I love dancing and dancing gives me that sense of spaciousness and creativity that are elements of the kinds of movement my heart is drawn to. Dance classes also satisfy some of the major barriers I feel toward healthy movement in the winter. I love that it is an indoor activity that still feels wild and free. Gyms suffocate me and suck the joy out of exercise for me. So during the winter months I have to choose indoor options that feel fantastic, that I willingly will trade my precious babysitter hours for.

Every single time I go to a dance class I beam from within. I come home and feel flexible, I feel lighter, and I feel happy and replenished. I'm more likely to keep the momentum going between dance classes with stretching, at home yoga positions, or energy mind-body movements each day. I'm more likely to bundle up and take trail walks when the weather allows once I've broken through the stagnation of the winter months. If I place enough dance classes into my month, I'm more likely to keep healthy movement going throughout the days in between.

So you first engage with your interests—tap into the deeper connection of movement and joy and take the essence of those visions and generate some stepping stones that are more within your reach in the life you live right now.

## Step 2: Start Where You Are

It may seem obvious (all the answers do once you hear them, right?) but many people jump right into goals around movement that are huge leaps beyond where they are right now. Some of us have strict definitions in our head around what a legitimate workout routine would consist of and feel like anything less is a waste of time. So let's take it a step back. Think again of that empty pool dry as a bone with all the hoses pointing in. If your hose of Joyful Movement is not turned on at all, even a trickle is an improvement. And from a trickle you can slowly and surely increase the volume until you get a flow going that feels perfect for your life and wellbeing. But many of us get stuck in that all or nothing place with movement. If we can't turn our hoses on full speed, we don't turn them on at all. Or we try to turn them on at full capacity only to realize the demands of our lives and schedules (or bodies themselves) can't sustain that kind of flow immediately, so we burn out fast. Keep your initial commitments simple. Set yourself up for massive success in this area. Guard against this becoming obligatory and a forced experience. The difference between true motivation versus sheer drudgery is connecting back to an honest sense of enjoyment.

I loved reading about a woman who was over one hundred pounds overweight. For years, she had tried diet after diet and exercise routine after exercise routine that never stuck and left her feeling more and more despondent. Then, one day, she decided she just wanted to have some fun again. She wanted to get out and live a little again. For this woman, the option to stay in her home for fear of feeling ashamed or awkward at a dance class felt more painful than missing out on feeling fully alive and connected to others. So she started going to dance. At first she would show up and all she could do was sway back and forth in the back of the room and enjoy the music. But she kept showing up. She did what she could. Her commitment was simply to get to that class once a week. She enjoyed the process. She connected with others and delighted in their expressions and movements. Every week she saw the tiniest of progress. She could keep up a few minutes longer before having to sit and rest. She could bend and sway a little further each time. Yes, it felt awkward and yes she had to battle a whole lot of internal messages that told her every reason she should quit, but this time she also had awakened something else within her. She had awakened the connection of movement to joy. She awakened the connection of movement to something that she personally enjoyed, to delight, to connection with others. Whether she was resting or swaying, she loved feeling a part of the class, she loved hearing the music, she loved seeing the smiles of the other women, and she felt better about herself every time she walked out of that dance studio. She was reconnecting her physical body with her emotional body and together they reinforced and replenished each other and it spurred her on. After a while, bit by bit, she was not only fully participating in the classes but she was going three times a week. But she didn't start there. She started where she was and she allowed her interest to lead her forward.

## Step 3: Keep It Simple

The simplest ways to move and love your body are often the most healing. One of the issues around Joyful Movement is that we overcomplicate it. We think we need expensive gym memberships or workout gear or high level training or the latest yoga mat technology before we can get started. By far, the best form of exercise is simply walking. Regardless of where you are in the world, you can get started by just walking through your front door. The other reason I love walking is that I am a big believer of connecting our movement with nature in as many ways as possible. Walking allows us to really feel our bodies as they are. It allows us to experiment with different levels of exertion. It can act as a conduit to allow our minds to shift gears, relax, and wander while our bodies are in motion. It engages the senses, you feel different sensations of the earth or ground under your feet, and you hear the sounds of the trees, birds, cars, chatter of people as you go by. You watch a changing landscape and get a larger horizon view of the sky in your field of vision, which is hugely healing to someone who feels stuck and suffocated in her life or mind.

When you consider turning on the hose of Joyful Movement, consider ways you can make the water flow with ease and delight. Let your body tell you how it wants to move and grow and expand in this core essential. From this place, you'll feel the ripples of benefit throughout your whole wellbeing.

## Your Brain on Movement

On a bright Saturday morning, I walked into a gorgeous room with vaulted ceilings, long stretches of open windows letting in natural light, gleaming wood floors, and richly colored brick walls. Just being in this space felt delightful. The teacher gathered us in a circle and welcomed us, sharing that we would be focusing on the concept of creativity for today's Nia dance class. She went on to share that what our bodies do, in the physical plane, creates corresponding neural pathways in our brains. When we move our bodies in new and unexpected ways, our brains have to get out of their old patterns and recreate new pathways as well. Just days before I had led a class on creating more calm, clarity, and creativity through training your brain to work differently and taught about these exact concepts. Now, though I stepped into the classroom as a student, I was given the chance to put my own teachings into practice and massage my brain in ways it hadn't been for months.

For many of us who struggle with being too much in our heads, and whose monkey brains are huge sources of stress, engaging in the regular practice of Joyful Movement is a powerful tool to restore and reset our mental and emotional wellbeing. In fact our bodies are meant to move through our emotional experiences. Moving our tissues helps process our emotions, it releases stress, it processes (and releases) trauma, it releases joy and gratitude. It's the ultimate connector and integrator for all the parts of who we are—when we give our bodies healthy movement it elevates our physical, emotional, mental, and spiritual health. Movement at its most elemental level is a bridge between our inner worlds and our outer worlds. When our inner worlds becomes tight and tense, when our emotions feel wound up and knotted, sometimes the easiest way to smooth them out is by leading the way with our bodies. There's never been a time in my life when I haven't felt emotionally better after getting some healthy movement in. And when I'm feeling most anxious, overwhelmed, and bottled up, that can often be the hardest times to get over the hump and give myself some time to get moving, but it's always the perfect remedy.

Remember how we talked about getting to calm from the back door when we explored our core essential of a Calm Mind? In the same way, when we feel down or blue we can overly retreat inward and this becomes a stagnant, congested way of living. Using our bodies to increase ease, expression, and flow is an elegant way to get our minds and moods unstuck as well. This is a fundamentally different way of thinking about our core need for Joyful Movement. Instead of considering how many miles we need to run, how to get our blood pressure in the right zone, or how to burn a certain amount of calories, we see moving our bodies like a de-tangler for a knotted up life. We can ask our bodies to bear the gifts of an uplifted mind and mood.

## Mini-Task Your To-Do List

Without a doubt, one of the biggest challenges I hear moms talk about in my community is their desire to get more healthy movement in. They share they have it on their priority lists week after week and it never gets done. I believe much of this is because we don't enjoy what we tell ourselves we need to do. So after working through the earlier parts of this chapter, I hope you start to consider types of movement that feel good to you that would make you feel happy and excited to prioritize. But nonetheless, even sometimes the most Joyful Movement ideas need extra strategies to get done.

I want to talk about how to make it happen, which is really a conversation about all the little barriers in the way. One of my favorite strategies to work through these barriers is to mini-task them. You may have on your list: "take a walk," but what's actually true about that line item is there are a series of mini-tasks that have to happen in order to make "take a walk" actually happen in your life. So the first step in mini-tasking is to break even the simplest task down into its smaller parts. Let's go through the goal of "take a walk for thirty minutes this week." In order to get that accomplished here are the smaller details that have to be worked through.

1. What day are you going to take a walk?
2. What time are you going to take a walk?
3. What are you going to wear?
4. Will you be doing this with someone else?
5. Where are you going to go?
6. Do you have open time in your day (will the kids be in school, will you take them along, or do you need a babysitter)?

All of these details need to be addressed if you are going to take that walk. Now once walking becomes a more regular part of your life, many of these details can be handled without thinking much about them. But in the beginning, they can act like major road bumps, keeping you from ever making progress. This is true for anything on your to-do list that never seems to get done. They often have hidden details within that haven't been addressed and are acting like friction, keeping you from accomplishing them. So in order to take that walk, you'll need to know what you're going to wear. In fact, I suggest the night before you lay out your workout clothes and sneakers so you can easily change into them if need be. Why not put a water bottle next to your clothes too? You'll need to look at your calendar and specifically pen in when you are going for the walk and coordinate if you need any support to have that time freed up. You'll want to think through if you want to reach out and walk with someone else or if you'd rather go alone. You'll want to think through where you are going to walk—around your neighborhood, at a park, at the mall?

I'm one of those list nuts who love to cross off what I've accomplished during the day. So what I've done with some of my difficult-to-accomplish goals is to write out every mini-task detail within in. Once I get that walk in, I've actually crossed off seven items on my list and I feel hugely productive. Make sure you chose movement that feels really good.  Make sure your goals are appropriate from where you start. Make sure you keep your goals simple, because even a very simple goal requires you to change habits. Make sure you identify all the mini-tasks within it that need to be dealt with. Then watch yourself move steadily forward on nourishing the core essential of Joyful Movement in your life.

## Inner Movement of Joy

Your body needs movement and activity, but so does your mood and mind. Our intellect, creativity, and self-expression can also feel stale and stagnant if they aren't engaged for long stretches of time. Similar to how the core essential of Restorative Rest had a deeper application as we considered ways our life needed to honor the natural ebb, the core essential of Joyful Movement has a deeper layer to consider as well. Our inner world needs to experience healthy flow, too.

I remember the first time I realized I'd lost the practice of creativity, self expression, and joy as a mother. I was about six months into motherhood and my mother showed up one afternoon unexpected to take my little one for an hour and give me a break. There I was, in an empty house with an hour of precious, glorious time to myself and I walked around in circles before I defaulted into cleaning up and getting toys organized. I sat there in the middle of the living room with toys in my lap and just cried. I hadn't realized how disconnected from myself I'd become. Life with little ones (and big ones) can fast become task-oriented and outward-focused. Preserving and incorporating activities that bring you fulfillment, creativity, and enjoyment can easily get lost in the shuffle, but they're equally crucial to our wellbeing.

Personal growth and creativity need movement in our lives as well. The best thing I did for myself in this area was to engage the partial solution strategy. Maybe I couldn't spend hours painting like I used to, but I could steal away a few minutes with colored pencils and a sketchbook from time to time. Maybe I couldn't travel like I used to, but I could still flip through gorgeous coffee table books, read travel articles and linger in the travel sections of Barnes and Noble. Maybe I couldn't stay out late nights listening to live music like I used to, but I could check out weekend bands in the park or update my iPod list with new songs. The point is to first reconnect with what your interests are, what lights you up, what you care about, what you enjoy doing and then find out-of-the-box ways to bring those elements into your life. Start with one, you don't have to have all your interests or passions represented … just start with one and build from there.

## The Mama Joy Strategies

I want to share a strategy that served me well when I felt devoid of any creative outlets in my daily life. Part of the challenge, I found, was the unpredictability of the "me" time that would open up. Not only did I often not know when those gaps would come in the week, I also never knew how long they'd last. So unless I was prepared, they were often squandered. To counter this I created a Mama Joy bag. I found a bag I wasn't using and claimed it for these little opening in my days and weeks. I stocked it full of things like essential oils, my journal and a pen, the latest book I was reading, a small sketch pad and colored pencils, my iPod and earphones, my travel bible, and a Mother's Wisdom deck. Sometimes I included simple art supplies or even our portable DVD player loaded with an indie documentary I'd wanted to watch. What was important was that I was ready, I anticipated times when I could engage in my own interests and creativity so when they opened up, I could grab the bag and go. Even if I stayed in the house, the bag kept my things organized and easily found. I've encouraged other moms to not only make a Mama Joy bag for themselves, but also to keep a running list of Mama Joy ideas of activities that make them happy, feel connected to their interests and kept them intellectually, emotionally and creatively fed.

The core essential of Joyful Movement is about how we engage the part of the ebb and flow of our lives which is the out-breath. Many times all our outer energy, time and resources are spent on caring for and tending to others' needs. Some of our internal resources need to be reserved for our own healthy movements and growth. As you care for this core essential in both body and mind, you'll find more vitality and vigor in your everyday life. This is the core essential that not only fills the well, but lights the flame so you begin to feel filled up and fully alive again. Here's a quick recap of the tools and strategies to get the core essential of Joyful Movement into your life.

## Joyful Movement Tool Box

- *Experiment with the Tropical Island Journal prompt*

- *Create a Delightful Movement Vision Board*

- *Choose activities that capture the essence of how you want to feel when you exercise*

- *Set realistic goals that honor where you're starting from*

- *Mini-Task your movement goals into all the smaller tasks that are involved*

- *Keep it simple and consider walking to get started*

- *Assemble a Mama-Joy bag to be ready for small openings in your day to bring in more creativity and self-expression*

# Chapter 7

# Anchored Quiet

Quiet is not a sound many of us hear throughout our days. And for some, quiet actually feels unnerving. We're so accustomed to a constant stream of stimulation we hardly notice the noise and distraction coming at us all day. Our brains are wired to pay attention to changes in the environment. TV's a great example that's tapped into this neurological response. The changing scenes, bright colors, and fast movements all keep us in an alert state—and we've become addicted to the stimulation. Biochemically, this alert state triggers the stress response which increases the adrenaline in our system all day long. Whenever we experience a lull in our days, we reach for something to turn on … we turn on music, we check our phone, we mentally review the litany of tasks ahead of us, we click on the TV just to hear the chatter of commercials from another room—anything to keep the low-level buzz going. Background noise makes us feel comfortable.

# Fragmented Mind, Fragmented Life

I've heard many women share that as soon as things get too quiet, their anxiety rises and they feel like they're about to crawl out of their own skin. I can relate. This is how meditation felt to me when I first began it. It's also how I felt when I began wanting to become more mindful in my daily life. For example, when I try to be present with my kids for a long stretch of time, I'm shocked at how hard it is for me to turn off the distractions—both external and internal—and simply be with the person right in front of me. My stress default is to escape and distract my mind rather than settle in and connect to the world and people around me. Before I even realize it, I can find myself checking my phone for alerts or hopping on the computer to look at my inbox. When we keep our minds chronically fragmented, we begin to live fragmented lives. It's like having cracks in the bottom of your pool. You never feel replenished because the water is seeping through all the places of distraction we've built into our days. I've heard from countless moms I work with they're experiencing significant amounts of A.D.D.-like symptoms in their life. Their minds feel scattered and frazzled. They have a hard time focusing and staying on task. They have a hard time slowing down, calming down and just being in the present moment. It's a growing epidemic among our children and adults alike.

We hail multitasking as a prized skill in our culture, but studies show it doesn't add up to greater productivity. In fact you may be able to do more than one thing at a time, but your brain actually can't focus on more than one thing at a time. Your mind can only give your attention to one thing at a time, so while it seems as though you're focusing on many things at once, your brain is actually toggling back and forth between multiple sources of stimuli many times a minute just trying to keep focused on all that's in front of you (or that's reaching you through your senses). Keeping ourselves always plugged in and surrounded by noise keeps our brains in a constant flux of scattered attention. It's not only exhausting to keep this up, but it diminishes our effectiveness and efficiency. Researchers have found when people are multitasking they make 50% more errors and they take 50% longer to get the tasks done.[10] Furthermore, your thinking brain has two major functions: one is to collect information; the other is to synthesis and process it. You simply cannot make wise choices or find creative solutions in your life if your brain is always firmly stuck in the receiving input mode. We need times to process and reflect. We need downtimes to make sense of it all and to sort through the static and chaos to find order and clarity.

While the arguments against living an over-booked life are many, for our core essential of Anchored Quiet we'll explore how we can begin to bring more times of quiet into our lives and the connection quiet has to our spirit's need for nourishment. We'll talk about the role quiet plays in hearing what's most important … and the role it plays in discerning what's not important. I've found while quiet is a basic requirement for our wellbeing, both physically and mentally, it's also the doorway through which we bring in wellbeing to our spiritual nature as well.

## What Has Access to You?

I want you to imagine there's a bubble all around you extending to about one foot outward from the center of your body in all directions. Now consider everything that penetrates your bubble and reaches your eyes and ears all day long. What's allowed access to you? Throughout your day be mindful of what is getting through and whether you want it to. Part of the challenge of working from home and owning my own business is the lack of inherent boundaries around work time and life time. It's been a particularly sensitive topic within my marriage since Mike is very aware of when I'm physically with the family, but mentally checked out—taking short trips to my office to check email or crafting ideas in my head for new articles or talks. I've found the key to having a well-integrated life is actually having well-established boundaries around my time. This is true not only for work-life balance for but for all of life balance as well.

A couple of weeks ago I was at the playground with my kids. It was an unusually warm spring day and this park had water sprays going in the middle; the kids were howling with delight. I settled on a grassy spot nearby with a good view and automatically grabbed my phone to check emails. Within minutes my phone went dead and I found myself outside on a soft grassy patch, under a gorgeous blue sky, in absolutely perfect weather … fidgeting and restless not knowing what to do with myself. While I don't have data to back this up, I can share from my own experience, plugging into technology all the time is a form of addiction. And unplugging makes you feel just as uncomfortable, antsy, and anxious as weaning off any other addiction would make you feel.

So I began to do the Five Senses Exercise to calm the rising squirminess inside. This exercise helps me whenever I'm starting to feel the need to escape or when the current situation I'm in feels irritating (think traffic, grocery lines, gearing up to play hair salon with your five year old for the tenth time of the day). The Five Senses Exercise helps me when I need to make the transition from being checked-out to checked-into my life. It's also a great one to do with your kids. Just ask them the questions out loud and let everyone spend a couple minutes quietly thinking of the answers in their own heads. Here's how you do it.

## The Five Senses Exercise

1. Always begin by taking a couple long deep nose breaths with closed eyes.
2. Now softly open your eyes and take a minute to soften your jaw, forehead and neck.

3. Work your way through each of the following questions. Focus on each sense giving yourself time to get as detailed an answer as possible. Keep the line of inquiry matter of fact. Without making judgments, simply name what is happening around you at this very moment.

- What do I see?
- What do I feel on my skin?
- What do I feel in my body?
- What do I hear?
- What do I smell?
- What do I taste?

This simple exercise brings you into the present moment. The more you can do this without emotional baggage attached to your observations, the more you can allow your here-and-now to be a perfect place to be. For example, let's say you're sitting in traffic. It's tempting to begin describing the lines of cars ahead of you with disdain and frustration. Instead try to simply describe the scene as if you were relating it to an artist on the phone, what details would she need in order to capture your frame of view on paper.

## Get Intentional With Your Time and Attention

This is a simple beginning way to bring Anchored Quiet into your day by becoming aware of the world around you, as it is. It carves out a space of time, even in the middle of busyness, to focus your attention on the present moment in a calm and peaceful way. As you begin to pay more attention to the noises and influences around you, be mindful of who and what has access to you. Consider carving out space in your days for tech-free time zones, where you unplug and turn off alerts from your phone or devices. Consider having TV free times or background noise-free times in your home to get reacquainted with spending time in your day without all the distractions. You'll also want to take assessment of who has access to you and whether your interactions with them are building you up or draining you out. We'll go into this concept more in the core essential, Authentic Connections.

The next step in establishing Anchored Quiet in our lives is to bring in intentional times of protected quiet into our days.

## Quiet

Quiet is food for my spirit. It's nourishment for my soul. When I go too long without eating food, my body starts to get shaky and weak, I have a hard time thinking straight. When I go too long without intentional times of quiet, receiving nourishment for my spirit, my heart gets shaky and has a hard time discerning the truth about who I am and the life around me. It's much easier for me to believe my life's a total mess when my heart is starving. After regular feasts of quiet, it's hard for me not to see the amazing abundance and goodness that's all around me.

Quiet cleans the lens through which I see my life. It calms the waters long enough for the muddiness to settle. When my core essential need for quiet is filled, I experience clarity and confidence. I'm grounded in an inner peace, even if my life whirls around me or the waves begin to rock the boat in a storm. When I think of being deeply replenished, having enough to meet the demands of my day, it's in the paradox of making space for openness that I'm most profoundly filled up.

## Make Space to Receive

I remember a short car trip we took as a family to my sister's house, about an hour away. At one point in the ride we had the radio on, the kids were sounding like a petting zoo in the back, and my husband and I were trying to carry on a conversation. Well, I started talking about a certain song I wanted him to remember. So I kept trying to hum the melody to the song, but I couldn't get it out. And after a couple failed attempts we both just looked at each other and burst out laughing at the absurdity of what I was trying to do.

Do you know how hard it is to sing a song when you have other competing songs in the background?

Here's the thing. Lessening the distractions and noise in my everyday life healed and nourished my emotional and mental health. But it also did something more. Quiet became a pathway for my heart to be cared for, healed and nourished. It's in my times of quiet that I hear God most clearly in my life and from that place, I can return to my everyday life anchored and peaceful. This is how I've come to understand it. During my times of quiet I began to actually "hear" something like a tone … as if a tuning fork was struck. Not so much in an audible way, but more in a sensory way.  I began to get familiar with what God's frequency felt like in my body and spirit. Instead of trying to think about God, I connected to the feeling of being close to God. I began to know the experience, the resonance, of having Truth and Love flowing in and around and through me. In fact the actual word universe comes from uni (one) and verse (song)— one song. It's tuning into the one song of all creation which comes from the mark of the one who created us. As a Christian, I meet Jesus in this still, quiet place. I know the women who'll be reading this book come from many varied backgrounds and belief systems … and yet, still, we all understand and know our spirit's need for renewal and refreshment. We each need the opportunity to be in stillness and quiet in order to create a refuge away from the world for our spirits to breathe. As Maya Angelou said, "There is a place in you that you must keep inviolate, a place that you must keep clean. A place where you say to any intruder, 'Back up, don't you know I'm a child of God.'" When we don't give ourselves times of Anchored Quiet, we can't protect that place within us which is sacred.

The more time I spent in Anchored Quiet, the more choices and decisions in my day to day life became easier. When I was in tune to God's frequency, I began to know whether something enhanced or diminished its frequency. That's how I came to understand and trust my divine intuition. First by connecting to the One who had the master note and then leading my life in a way that kept that note amplified. Either things in my life fit into the rhythm or caused dissonance.

When you study the power and beauty of our brains, there's amazing evidence the practice of quieting your thinking mind is actually good and necessary for all the parts of your whole-person health. If you watched your brain on an EEG during deep prayer or meditation this is what happens: all the typical neural pathways that light up your frontal "thinking" lobes begin to dim and slow down. This is called frontal deregulation. When your thoughts are given a chance to rest, the back parts of your brain can begin to light up and explore new ways to connect and integrate all the information you take in all day long. The way I see it, God has designed us to literally open up new ways of understanding ourselves, our lives, our challenges, and our solutions when we honor His command to "Be still and know that I am." Instead of emitting beta waves like we do when our frontal cortex is hopping all day long, in times of stillness, quiet, and meditation, we release alpha waves from our brains. Producing alpha waves promotes an overall sense of relaxation, ease, and calm. I've experienced all of this as a result of prayerful meditative time. As mothers we are nurturers and intuits, givers and menders, creatives and doers ... we need to open spaces in our lives to be deeply connected to our hearts, to our callings, to our divine guidance, because it equips us with a greater capacity to be present and serve more deeply.

Quiet. There's no other way around it. We cannot begin to see clearly into our own lives when the noise is too loud around us. Protecting time and space in our days for quiet, reflection, prayer, meditation, inspiration, processing … it's just so crucial on every level. I have many blind spots, we all do. We need to keep our spirits connected to a higher, wiser, grander source. And so, this core essential of true replenishment is about becoming more fully present to your life and to the presence of the divine in your life through the practice of quiet. And when we enter into this still place within, what we find is Love which, of course, is the greatest healer of all.

## Let Love In

One summer I spent a few months in Tanzania, East Africa working at a small school in a rural village, teaching English as well as cleaning and repairing the buildings. One of the days I spent volunteering at a local Mother Teresa's orphanage there. Sometime around mid-day when lunch was about to be served, I found myself in the back corner room where there were just a couple children. The Sister in charge was getting ready for lunch and asked me if I would feed one of the boys. Of course, I would. Yes.

I cannot remember his name, which kills me because this is one of the sharpest, clearest heart memories I have in my life. He was about fifteen years old. And he was severely handicapped. He was tall, but since his arms and legs were crippled, he was long and curled. His neck permanently stuck in an upward thrust. He had a hard time controlling his tongue, so feeding him needed to be slow and careful. I sat on the floor and we arranged him to lay across my lap, with his head cradled in my left arm. I slowly fed him oatmeal and lovingly held his glance the whole time. I wish I could show you his eyes. They were the largest, brightest, deepest, most grateful eyes I've ever seen. I could hardly handle the ache that collapsed my heart. As we gazed at each other, I had an open smile and tears kept rolling down my face. I'd never experienced anything like this before.

He didn't seem to feel awkward that I was smiling and crying and fumbling with his food. He just lay in my arms, with the most beautiful eyes I've ever seen, gracing me with his gratitude and love for being there with him. After lunch, I was a bit on emotional overload and needed some breathing space so decided once he, (can we just call him Matthew so he has a name as I tell you this?) once Matthew laid down for a nap, I moved into the room with all the infants.

One of the most pressing needs for visiting volunteers is to just hold these babies. Because, while the sisters can keep them clean and fed, there are just too many babies and the sisters couldn't possibly hold them all for the amount of time a human baby deserves, needs, to be held every day. So I just picked up these babies and walked with them and snuggled and whispered prayers into their necks and kissed their heads and rocked myself to calm as I held them close and breathed in their beauty.

About ten years after that summer work trip, I would become a mother myself. I think back to that day often. I had no idea at the time that I experienced a glimpse of the depth it takes to really love someone. A glimpse of what you get when you choose to let love come pouring through into the awkwardness, the brokenness, the imperfections, the ugly, and the difficult. It was my first glimpse at what you receive when you love the hard to love—and that really there is no hard to love—once you make the choice to love, it's all easy. It wasn't hard to love Matthew ... what was hard was to soften into the experience, to be there, truly be there—to let my tears come streaming down even though I felt self conscious and uncomfortable.

In my everyday life, when I'm so caught up in my head and my to-dos and the busyness and my need to control the day, I find myself resisting when my kids look "ugly." When they have attitude. When they're fresh. When they aren't listening. When they're rude or arrogant. When the level of chaos is giving me heart palpitations and I think I'm going to fly into code red. I often don't soften; I try to control and force everything back into order again. Matthew wasn't able to mask his needs—he was bare to the world. Just like the infants I held and rocked. Like my own children when they were babies. And now as they grow and assert themselves, I get tricked into thinking they are not deserving of my compassion, my love, when they are at their roughest. I get tricked into thinking they aren't needy of my love exactly when it feels hardest to give it. I think love has a whole lot to do with cleaning up your own heart so that you can have the courage to meet someone where they are. That's what my times of anchored quiet do for me—they clean up my own heart.

We're all needy. We're all difficult. We all have rough edges and scratchy spots that don't feel good to rub up against. We all struggle with doubt and guilt, with anxiety and insecurity. No mom is insulated from being torn to pieces sometimes over how crazy hard this path really is. What if instead of wishing ourselves to be different we loved our own broken parts? What if we actually opened up to the One who could heal the broken parts and remind us of who we really are, who we're really becoming? What if we didn't spend all our energy trying to hide the ugly parts of ourselves, trying to be the perfect mother, the one who never needs or asks or requests for anything? What if we started instead to show up, fully and honestly, in quiet spaces in the light of the One who can give us all we need, can fill the spaces in our spirit we long to have filled? I think it would look like radiance. For me, choosing grace looks like a softening into love. A softening into being loved, even when (most especially when) I'm at my neediest, which is often when I'm at my ugliest.

When softening into love becomes our default response in life, we get to experience a fountaining over of love. The core essential of Anchored Quiet gives us this space within that allows grace and love to take deep roots in our lives. Without this core essential we may set out to build gorgeous lives but they are set on quicksand and as soon as the demands of life come in, we have no anchor to hold on to. That's what cultivating a practice of Anchored Quiet has done in my life, so let's explore more deeply how to bring anchored quiet into our very full (and noisy) days.

## 3 Steps to Bring Quiet In

How can you commit to some soul-silence time every day? Some not-busy-doing time? How can you strengthen the skills of listening and reflecting, observing and processing when we live in such a reactive, loud, and distractible culture? How can you turn off the noise just a bit?

I know that for some of you, that feels like a slap in the face kind of question. It isn't because you don't want quiet time that you don't have it. It's because of where you are in life and the demands on you from the moment you wake to the time you sleep that squeeze out the opportunity for the stillness you crave. I get that to my bones. From wherever you are right now in life your goal is not to jump to the other side of the river in one fell swoop. Your job is to look for the closest stepping stone to where you are standing and begin there.

Perhaps, for you, that can only be five minutes every day. And maybe those five minutes are stolen away behind a locked bathroom door. Regardless of what your first baby-step goal is toward prioritizing and bringing times of quiet and reflection into your day, I want you to be intentional about it. Consider the tools we'll explore in this chapter and make a plan for using those few precious minutes wisely in a way that reflects your true desire for self and spirit level connection. This is how this process looks like in reality:

## Step 1: Commit and show up.

Commit some time every day to the practice of finding that space to hear the tuning fork. In this way you're getting familiar with your spirit's tone. For some this can simply be following your breath in and out for five, ten or fifteen minutes every day. It's a chance to unplug your thinking mind and give it respite from the noise. For others, this can be a time to open your heart to God's presence. I've often struggled with trying to understand God, sorting through dogma and doctrine, coming to terms with confusing thoughts and doubts. What I've found is when I simply show up and meet God in this still place within; there is no need for words. I don't need to worry about details or explanations or definitions. I can simply be with God and feel His presence within me. It's like knowing the voice of your lover … or even more intimately, knowing the nuance of how your lover writes, how he laughs, the curve of his handwriting, the choice of his words, the shade of his humor.

In the beginning as I was nurturing myself back from a place of intense depletion, my times of quiet were really just me showing up. For a long stretch, my prayer times were flooded with tears. I would sit cross legged, head hanging, and shoulders slumped. I'd just say, "God, I need to feel your love. I just need more of you." I would sit in the front window of our living room, right where the sun came streaming through. I imagined divine love pouring down on me. Elemental and simple. Truthfully, I had nothing more to give or say. One of the blessings of feeling depleted is you start to finally get out of your own way. You can just be present and open. These "I'm literally just showing up" kinds of prayer carved out a space within me that used to be chaotically filled with requests and questions, affirmations and worries. Once I started just knocking on the door, sliding onto the sofa, and resting my head on His shoulder without saying much of anything, a whole new understanding of the power of quiet changed my life.

The biggest hurdle is simply the commitment of the time. What matters more than the length of time you reserve is the consistency of having that time daily. Consider setting out a goal for yourself for one month. Every day, choose a certain amount of time that you will protect for Anchored Quiet. Whether its five minutes or fifty minutes, it matters more that you do it daily. This practice deepens and ripens over time.

## Step 2: Listen for the God-Frequency in Your Everyday Life.

Step 2 is experiencing this sacred connection of your spirit even in the midst of your day. It's about finding the extraordinary laced among the ordinary. Step 2 is when you begin to hone in and trust your divine intuition to direct you throughout your day and begin to align your outer world with your inner world. The more time we spend connected to our sacred center, the greater the buffer zone we create between the outside noise of the world and interior voice of truth. Self care and spirituality are inseparable to me. In fact, when we talk about an integrative life, connecting with the divine is the thread that binds all the parts of our lives into a whole. Just like a muscle, the more time I spend reconnecting to my center, the more I feel God's guidance in my everyday life, synchronicities and serendipity become a normal part of my day.

## Step 3: Record and Account Your Experiences.

When you see the light reflected around you, when you get an intuition hit, when you hear the sacred tone of truth even while the noise is all around you, it's essential to record and keep account. One of the most powerful things we can offer to ourselves and our children is to be the protector and passer-on of our stories. There's power when you record it, preserve it, have something to read over and remind yourself of. It enhances your life and makes you keener and sharper to seeing the breadcrumbs along the trail leading you on. The other reason recording is essential is because what we record amplifies.

Time and space, memory and attention are funny things in this universe. We think they're linear and static but they aren't. We're living in a universe that's like a fun house. Think about those twisted bent mirrors you always find in the clown houses at carnivals. Just like the curves of the mirror that make the image bigger, what you put your attention on in life ends up increasing in your life. If you want more peace, blessings, and clarity, then record what you have in your life right now—keep your focus on those things and more will follow.

There's also something powerful about engaging your senses. Writing, thinking, reading, speaking, and visualizing are magnifying glasses. And here's the thing—you're already doing these things. It isn't a case of whether or not you use these tools. You're always thinking, speaking, and visualizing—it's how your mind is wired to make sense of the world. When we begin to intentionally record the good around us, the guidance we've received, the graces, and the insights—we impress our new stories into our subconscious and we'll become more skilled at seeing the good, the guidance, the grace, and the insights that come to us every day.

## Ways to Spend Anchored Quiet Time

Now that you're carving out protected time each day for Anchored Quiet, how do you fill that time? At first, I knew I needed quiet but I'd often feel like I was jumping out of my head just sitting still. Here are three ideas to get you started.

## • Meditation or Contemplative Prayer

Renee Trudeau, a leading expert in life-balance and mother's wellness, and a dear friend of mine, recently told me about Father Thomas Keating's work on contemplative prayer.[11] As I read his book, Open Mind, Open Heart, I realized that I'd been doing this kind of meditation for many years now. I simply didn't know there was a whole movement behind it! Contemplative prayer is essentially holding a single word or image in your mind which represents for you your intention to connect your spirit with the Divine Spirit. As other thoughts come into your mind, and they will, you simply allow them to float away as if on a river, without any attachment. I love how Fr. Thomas explains, you can't control your thoughts from floating by like boats, but you can choose not to climb aboard. So instead of trying to rid your mind of thoughts during this time, you simply disengage from them. When you recognize them, you can return to your word or image to return to relaxing into spending quiet, open time in God's presence.

Another simple meditation is to use your breath as the anchor that you return to as you allow your thoughts to settle down and quiet. As you sit quietly, if you become aware of a thought in your mind, simply release it and allow it to float along its way by bringing your focus back to where your breath and following it on its path in and out of your body.

## • Calming or Binaural music

I also love to use the tool of calming music—most especially music with binaural beats designed to guide your brain into producing alpha waves. Many benefits have been studied in connection with these positive brain patterns including heightened focus, expanded creativity, better pain control, and enhanced learning capacity.[12] When you can support your mind to relax more fully into the alpha wave state, it becomes much easier to still your body and mind at a deeper level.

• Guided meditations to relax and calm body and mind

Many people enjoy guided meditations which talk you through calming and relaxing each part of your body. This is a wonderful way to encourage your physical body to release the tension and stress its holding, so as you open into a deeper place of silence in your thoughts and heart. A guided mediation can be tremendously helpful if your body feels tense or antsy when you try to quiet your mind.

## Ways to Record and Amplify

Often after my times of quiet, I am filled with inspiration, truth and messages of wisdom. Here are some recording strategies I employ to help me capture the gems that surface from my times of quiet.

• Rambling Pages

I have a special notebook that I call my Rambling Pages. It's not my usual journal, or my sketch book, or a place to jot down to-do reminders. Inspired by what Julia Cameron calls morning pages from her famous book, The Artist's Way, I use this book to help me process thoughts that are not completely formed or intentional or even reflective, but that need to be expressed. Many times I'll grab my Rambling Pages journal before my times of quiet- especially when my mind is already wound up and racing. It helps me to get my incoherent thoughts out on paper to clear a way for me to enter a time of stillness.

Here's how it works. Open a blank page and write. Anything. All things. The key is to write whatever bubbles up or floats across your mind, just keep writing. If you feel like stopping, make something up in order to keep the pen going. The key to this practice is to keep your writing fluid and in motion in order to allow the thoughts to come out as they surface. If you stop and think about what to write, you have now entered a different state and are no longer opening the channel to your inner, more random, more deeply rooted thoughts. This book should make no sense in normal journal terms. It may contain things you are embarrassed about, would never want another person to read, don't really feel or think, or are disjointed and hard to understand. That's the point. This is a place just to get some stuff out of your head.

## • Prayer Journal

Writing out your prayers is powerful. Not only do I use my journal to write out prayers from my perspective, I sometimes find myself writing a response from God's perspective. It's like His voice is coming through my heart and responding to me right in the pages of the journal as I write. I'll often simply ask a question and then pause. When I feel something responding within me I start to write it out. Of course, I never really know if it's God or me … but I've stopped worrying about that as much. If I trust God lives within me, I trust He's working in and through and around me all the time. Why can't He use my mind and heart to respond to me through my journal? I've been surprised by how much closer I feel in prayer when I allow my prayers to be written and reflected in this way.

## • Prompt-Led Journaling

I was first introduced to this kind of journaling when I took an online course by Andrea Scher called Mondo Beyondo.[13] Daily prompts were sent by email and I reserved some time everyday to reflect on them and write out my insights and responses. I've found whether you're a beginner journaler or more experienced, having some prompts to steer your thoughts into whole new rooms of discovery is a fantastic experience—especially if, like me, you tend to get into mental ruts and go over the same issues again and again. Reflective prompts give you new starting places to explore that break up negative patterns and open new ways of thinking about things. I was so impacted by this course, I created a course of my own for moms who want to explore the barriers in their lives that keep them from living their most vibrant lives called Vibrant Living Strategies. This has proved to be one of my most popular courses and I love witnessing the personal growth that happens when a mama gives herself a little time, paper and a pen.

• Gratitude Journal

Gratitude journals are focused on naming and counting the things you're thankful for in your life. Ann Voskamp is a leading voice for the power of gratitude in your life through her book (and online movement) called One Thousand Gifts.[14] I still have my gratitude journal from the months right before I met my husband. It reminds me of a time when I had both deep yearnings for things I didn't have yet (a family) and a heart full of gratitude for all the gifts I did have in my life. I find whenever I'm tipping the scales toward wanting more of what I don't have versus enjoying what I do have, a gratitude practice is strong medicine.

## How to Remember Your Song in Your Everyday

• The Heart Pause

What happens when you're in the thick of your day, the noise around you is rising, and you're having a hard time connecting to the still, quiet, spirit place within you? This is one of my very favorite tools to reach for in those moments. As soon as you recognize you need to reconnect, pause from whatever you are actively doing. Close your eyes, if you're able, and put your hand over your heart. In fact do it right now. Take thirty seconds, put down this book. Close your eyes, put your hand on your heart, and take a few calm breaths. Imagine all the energy that is scattered out in the world coming back to you and returning into your heart space. Can you feel your own sacred core getting stronger and more in focus? So often, what happens is that all day long we spread our core life energy all over the world—we give it out all day long—in our interactions and our busyness. From time to time, just the simple act of calling your energy back to yourself and taking a pause to focus inwardly toward your heart is very healing.

## Self Care and Spirituality

Something will happen as you commit to hearing your spirit's song in your life. You'll have to deal with the fear voices that rise up and try to make you smaller than you truly are. I hear all the time among the women I serve the inner conflict they feel around making changes and choices in their lives that would expose a brighter, happier, more fulfilled woman in the world. We begin to question whether it's selfish or greedy to focus on ourselves and the core essentials of our wellbeing. As we begin to trade the noise and distraction for quiet and calm, we wonder, "Who am I to want a different way of living? Is it okay that I am choosing to say no to certain things in order to protect my own wellbeing? Isn't it noble to sacrifice to a point where I give every last drop?"

It's a tricky thing talking about self care to mothers. Something happens when we cross over the motherhood threshold that radically changes the terrain of our lives. It's called sacrifice. We enter lives of self-sacrifice like we have never known before. Our lives are now tethered to another in a way that requires a level of self-sacrifice most of us happily, willingly, and completely sign up for. As my children's mother, I want to sacrifice for them. But sacrifice has become a confusing issue for modern mothers. On one hand we're culturally (and I believe genetically) designed to fully and whole-heartedly accept the walk of sacrifice in order to reap the tremendous benefits and joys of motherhood. On the other hand, we're chastised not to lose ourselves in the name of mothering. To reclaim a strong sense of who we are and prioritize our self care as non-negotiable.

My take? It's a farce that self-sacrifice and self-care are pitted against one another. The more I spend in quiet, the clearer it is to me my greatest purpose is to become the vibrant, beautiful, bright, and fulfilled woman God created me to be. My staying in a depleted, frazzled state of life was is in no way reflecting the grandeur, grace, or greatness of my creator. I believe there's a sweet spot where we hold both sacrifice and self care in our hands and this is where God's song is strongest in our lives. It's when we are living from our zone of thriving.  A mothering life rich in both self-sacrifice and self-care has built in harmony. They're natural checks and balances for each other. It's when one becomes dominant to the other that things get radically off kilter.

When you've experienced an imbalance of far too much self-sacrifice with very little self-care, you aren't self-sacrificing any longer, you're now firmly in the zone of self-neglect. My dear friend and manager for WellGrounded Life, Bren, shared with me that she's often reminded by a friend of hers that God doesn't require "burnt sacrifices." It isn't necessary for us to grind ourselves to the nub in order to do the great work of mothering. Is sacrifice required? Yes. But an unchecked life of sacrifice where we don't extend the same love and care to ourselves that we do to others isn't sustainable. On the flip side, when we move past self-care into self-absorption, that no longer truly replenishes us either. Self absorption diminishes our healthy growth. The best way to get a clear sense of where you're landing on the spectrum is in times of Anchored Quiet. When we quiet to noise around us, we can check in and get an honest pulse on where we need to shift to find the vital balance between caring for ourselves and caring for others. Let's review all the ways we discussed to enhance the core essential of Anchored Quiet in our days.

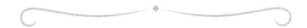

## Anchored Quiet Tool Box

- *Pay attention to what has access to you all day long; the people, sounds, and distractions that make their way into your "bubble"*

- *Practice the Five Senses Exercise when you are feeling the urge to check out of your here and now*

- *Protect times of quiet daily—regardless of how long you have, try to reserve some time everyday*

- *Meditate using your breath as your focal point*

- *Explore Contemplative Prayer as a form of meditation*

- *Use calming or binaural music to guide your brain into producing alpha waves*

- *Use guided meditation audios to help relax your body*

- *Record the insight or inspiration you experience from your times of quiet*

- *Find the ways God's song shows up in your everyday life*

- *Journal in one or more of these ways: Rambling Pages, Prayer journaling, Prompt-led journaling, or Gratitude journaling*
- *Practice the Heart Pause throughout your day*

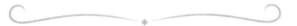

# Chapter 8
# Authentic Connection

My grandmother used to say "Show me your friends and I'll show you who you are." The more I learn about the way our brains are wired, the more her simplistic saying is spot on. We truly become like those around us. It's how we're designed to work. We all have what are called mirror neurons laced through our brains.[15] These neurons are special because they fire up both when we do a particular action and when we observe someone else doing that action. Whether we're the ones doing it or simply observing another person doing it, the same neuron will light up in your brain. So the neurons that fire when you smile are the same ones that fire when you observe someone else smile. If all you observed was that mirror neuron in someone's brain, you couldn't tell whether he was smiling or simply watching someone else smile—in the brain it's all the same.

## We're Becoming Like Those Around Us

This very powerful mechanism allows humans to experience empathy. When we observe the facial expressions of another person, the same neurons of our brain are fired up as if we ourselves had made that subtle facial expression. Our brains remember how we were feeling when we've made that facial expression before and then we can understand and empathize with the person we're observing. Women have more mirror neurons in our brains. It's in our nature to want to model the subtle feelings, beliefs, thoughts, actions, and expectations of those we come into contact with— and this all happens subconsciously. In fact, it's written into our physiological make up to use others as guideposts for our own growth. It's extremely difficult to establish your own positive personality and mood when you're constantly surrounded by people who model back negative personalities and moods. There's simply no denying who I surround myself with radically impacts who I'm becoming. So when I was working on replenishing my whole self—body, mood, mind and spirit—I looked at the people in my life and the impact they had on me.

When women make huge changes happen in their lives, especially when they've had difficulty in the past meeting their goals, they all have one essential element a part of their success: they've found their inner hut circle. On the Real Women Talking website this quote caught my eye, "You're not only in my village, you're in my hut."[16] To raise a child, it takes a village, and it's equally true to keep a mom healthy takes a village as well. And the people who fill your inner hut are crucial not only to your wellbeing but also to the trajectory of who you're becoming.

The truth is, modern society—which is often fast-paced, stressed-out and isolating—doesn't help us live the vibrant, happy, energized, and self-connected life most of us desire. Most of us watch each other through screens, where we post highlight reels of our lives on Facebook and Pinterest, but we lack the authentic whole-person connections that are crucial for our well being. Gathering your inner hut circle, then, is having critical relationships present in your life that support you toward becoming more fully who you are and spur you toward growing in the ways you want to grow. As I've reflected on my own inner hut relationships throughout my life, I've come to see three kinds of critical connection are present when I'm doing my best. Let's explore them a little more.

# Three Types of Inner Hut Connections

## 1. Soul-Sister Connections

Often you don't know what you need until you don't have it. This was certainly true for me when I became a new mother. I was living in New Jersey after spending eleven years living in California and Boston, where I was going to school. Soon after I moved back, I got married and had my first child, but my best friends were still scattered all over the country. At first, I did a pretty good job of keeping in touch with them. Our friendships were vital and close even though we were living so far away. I felt loved, supported, and filled up in this area.

But when I was catapulted into a whole new world of new motherhood, the lack of having close friendships nearby felt intense and painful. I came to realize very quickly the need I had for Soul-Sister connections. Now to be sure, I don't believe this looks the same for every one of us. What counts as a Soul-Sister connection for me will look very different for other women, but the essence of these connections most of us can relate to on some level.

Soul-Sisters are the women in our lives who bring in the laughter, sit with us when we're coming apart, normalize our craziness and give us perspective, because they love us for who we are, know us for who we are and can connect deeply with where we are in life—right in the here and now. In my life, I had the distinct feeling of lack in this area and I felt lost and very lonely, even though I was surrounded by people who loved me. Most of the women I work with who also feel the pang of loneliness without true Soul-Sister friendships in their life wish they could make these connections happen on demand, like ordering the perfect shoes from a mail-order catalog. I know I would have paid for a magic wand that produced these relationships in my life when I needed them most, but the reality is, sometimes we simply have to wait until they naturally happen in our lives. Later in this chapter, I'll talk about some strategies that are helpful if you don't feel you have the kind of Soul-Sister connections you yearn for right now in your life.

## 2. Mentor Connections

The second type of connection we all need is Mentors. These are other women in our lives who are the wise voice of perspective, advice, and encouragement. Now, of course, sometimes our Soul-Sisters also act as our Mentors, but sometimes these roles are filled by different people, too. Regardless of whether one person fills multiple roles for you, the lack of having one of these roles filled in your life leaves you diminished in some way. Many of us may have the mentor role in our own families—it could be our mother, our aunts, our sisters, our grandmothers—but many of us feel we're doing this alone, with very little guidance.

One of the things I love about the international community of vibrant moms I'm growing through WellGrounded Life is the reality that while many of the moms come into the fold wanting to take a class with me, they quickly find the gold hidden in the incredible community of women they have access to. It's amazing to watch moms come together from all over the world and play out Soul-Sister and Mentor roles for each other while establishing deep bonds of friendship. A while back, I began to strongly feel the need for a mama mentor in my own life. So I reached out to Kristin, a woman who'd been part of my community and taken my courses from my very first offering. I knew her as a friend over the years and knew her heart and her perspective on mothering. She was also just one step ahead of me in her family season. A mom of four, her youngest was the same age as my oldest. So I knew she'd still intimately remember what I was going through, but be just enough ahead of where I was to offer a different level of insight and wisdom.

When we have our mama-mentor calls we talk about what's on my heart and what's happening with the kids. She listens and asks questions. She shares her experiences and what's worked for her. She gives me a big-picture perspective which calms me and helps me keep little things little without drowning in my own struggles of the moment. In so many ways, Kristin enriches my life. Having some structure and intention around our conversations reminds me I can get wise perspective and support when I feel confused around mothering challenges. I can allow the messiness to be there because I know I've built-in checkpoints and times when I'll reflect on what's working and not working along the way.

If you don't have this kind of inner hut member in your life, try to brainstorm about someone you know (even casually) who you could ask if they'd be open to talking with you periodically as a mama-mentor. You could get together over the phone, on a walk, or over a cup of coffee once a month or so. For decades these kinds of relationships formed informally and fluidly across generations passing on wisdom, support and confidence from one mother to another. In today's society we often have to seek out these kinds of relationships, but they're crucial to our own capacity to mother well with inner peace and authentic connection.

## 3. Visionary Connections

Finally, a third critical role in our inner hut circle is the Visionary. These are people (or a person) in your life who hold the vision of who you're becoming and mirror back to you your best self, most especially when you feel lost as to who that woman is anymore. You know you have someone in your Visionary role when you feel lighter, taller, and happier to be with yourself after time spent with her. You remember who you are. Very often we can get into stuck places and our growth can feel stagnate. The people who hold the role of Visionary ignite excitement about change and growth. Their presence in our world helps us dream a little bigger and see a little farther into what's possible. At many crossroads in my journey, I've specifically sought out support from others to hold this space for me and help me wrap details around the fuzzy dreams I held in my heart. I lean into others for visionary support in my growth spiritually, personally, and professionally.

When these three roles are filled in some capacity, the Sister-Soul, the Mentor and the Visionary, my inner hut feels robust. I feel deeply supported and I'm bolstered in my capacity to do the tremendous work of mothering day in and day out. Like I've mentioned before, this has nothing to do with the number of people in your inner circle, but the quality of connections you have. Sometimes it may be just one other person in your life who offers you all of these connections, other times it's a constellation of friends and family who do the trick, but the lack of these critical connections can feel crippling because we're not meant to go through this alone.

## The Role of Your Spouse

My husband, Mike, is many things to me. He's my soul-level best friend, my deepest lover, and my comrade in this grand parenting journey. There's simply no one in the world that makes me laugh like he does. He offers me wisdom and perspective. No one sees me like he does, no one believes in me like he does, no one stands up and fights for me to become the best and brightest version of myself than he does. And yet, what I've found is things start to fall apart when I expect Mike to be my only source for these critical relationships.

Your spouse can be a very special part of your inner hut, but he cannot be all things for you. In fact, it's only when I began to circle myself and fill the core essential of Authentic Connections with other women and mothers in my life that my marriage relationship could truly blossom and grow into what it is today. While your husband can fill many roles in your life—there are some roles only he can (and should) fill. When I allow others to be a part of my inner hut circle, I'm replenished in my needs for core connection and I come to our marriage feeling full and alive. I can offer more of myself to him in the ways that he only gets to have. He feels the freedom of loving a woman who's not excessively needy or depleted and our relationship thrives.

My husband and I were only three months married when we became pregnant with our first child.  Still reeling in the bliss of being newlyweds, that excitement and energy quickly flowed into the dreams of starting a new family. We were still "babies" at this marriage thing when we become parents. I never thought much about the toll children take on a marriage. In abstract ways before becoming a mom, I imagined it would be a process of self-sacrifice that you would go through as you become responsible for another life, but I never thought about how children challenge the dynamic of your marriage relationship. I believe at the core of a true marital love is deep generosity. The decision to love this other person in our thoughts, words, and actions even when the feelings aren't there. Even when you're tired and selfish. When you're busy and overwhelmed. When you have your own ideas of where you want your life to head. At all these hundreds of moments every day you're given the opportunity to show up and see your spouse as his own person who's also growing and evolving.

You have the choice to know him more fully and support him in his walk. I'm in awe of my husband, of who he is and who he's becoming. And when I lose that awe, I lose the magic, every time. But now, with children, I've never felt so needy. So stretched beyond my capacity. So exhausted from giving and giving. So aware of my own limitations and pride. So tapped out.

And it's at this point I find myself most challenged in staying generous, compassionate, and loving toward my husband. I want to become a child myself again and scream I NEED … I WANT … ME ME ME. When the hoses have run dry for so long, I've shifted from sacrifice into self neglect and I feel hostile toward my spouse having any needs of his own. Generosity is the farthest thing from the natural leaning of my heart. This makes me think about the big horn sheep. Big horn sheep live on the slopes of steep mountains. They traverse these mountains on razor thin paths etched all around the mountain sides. They also cannot walk backward, only forward. So what happens when two sheep are walking along the same path in opposite directions and bump face first into each other? If they fought, one would surely die as he would have to be thrown from the path. They cannot walk backward and the path is far too thin for both to be on at once. The only option is for one to lie down. The other, then can cross on top, leaving both unscathed, safe, and ready to continue on their way.

When I feel that tightness rise up in me and I want to lash out and demand that my needs be cared for in my marriage, I'm often reminded of the big horn sheep. If I give myself time to settle down and be honest, I can calm the raging storm inside that says I have to demand and fight for my own way and force my needs to be taken care of. I can gain some perspective and realize that demanding from him what isn't reasonable for him to give me will only result in both of us being tossed off the mountain. Sometimes the act of caring for myself and reaching out for authentic connections that feed and replenish my soul is a way of loving my husband and honoring our marriage.

## Allow the Open Spaces

So by now, I hope I've convinced you of how crucial it is to have very specific kinds of relationships in your inner hut circle. But what happens when you don't have those people in your life yet? What to do with the empty spaces was one of my biggest (and hardest) learning curves yet.

Soon after the birth of my first child, I struggled with depression, in the depths of sleep-deprived neurosis that would give way to intense bouts of weeping at any moment. One of my clearest memories was one of the lowest, most broken points in that early journey. About two or three weeks after the birth of my son, my stitches hadn't come out from my episiotomy and I was feeling pain in that area so I thought I might have been infected. I made an appointment with my midwife (with whom I had a horrible experience with during the birth.) I sat in her examination room waiting to see her, holding back tears and desperately trying to keep it together. I was naked underneath a simple paper covering. It was cold in her office. I was slightly shivering.

She entered and never once looked me in the eyes. Speaking into her chart, she asked, "What's going on?" I told her that I was concerned about the stitches and that I felt sore in that area. She told me to lay back and barely touched me. "Everything looks fine. Anything else?" she asked. I said no. She left and closed the door. It must have taken me fifteen minutes to get myself composed from hysterically crying in order to dress and leave the building. I felt so unsupported, so abandoned, so uncared for I was stunned with pain.

But here's the interesting part of the story. I had a long history of difficulty and disappointment with this woman. I switched to her care when I was six months pregnant and as I was getting closer to delivery, even though I didn't feel good about the ways she interacted with me, how she answered my questions, the tone of her presence during the visits, I convinced myself I couldn't switch providers again at such a late time in the pregnancy. Things with her did not get better at the birth either. Gratefully, I had a doula who was with me and supported me through a very long labor, but the presence and intrusion of the midwife's attitude deeply affected me, not only while it was happening, but still to this day, I can feel a knot of resentment in my body rising. So I clearly had a history of bad experiences with this woman. And yet, I still continued to seek out her help and support. I still went to her as a source of the care, understanding, wisdom, and support I so desperately needed as a new mom as I was feeling like my life was capsizing around me.

I can remember the most curious experience happened that day somewhere between my hysterical crying in the office and when I reached my car in the parking lot. By the time I opened my car door and sat inside, an otherworldly peace saturated my whole being. I wasn't stuck in the hysteria and sadness that was swirling in head any longer, I simply felt calm. I felt held. I felt viscerally protected and cared for. I knew that I was all right. That I didn't need her, I could release her completely. I look back and know this moment marked a turning point in my own growth journey, a long, winding journey back to myself.

Sometimes the first step in circling yourself with the life-giving relationships you desperately desire is to clearly protect yourself from the life-sucking ones. In that moment, I began to understand that while I deeply needed authentic connections around me, I was okay with waiting for the right relationships to fill those voids rather than trying to fill those empty spaces with people who were not worthy of them. The first step in circling your life with authentic connections, then, is to choose to have open space around you ready for the right people to come close rather than trying to fill those spaces with people who do not serve you well.

As I drove home after that appointment, I was calmer than I had been for a long time. It was a gorgeous late October day. The sun was strong and warm in a clear blue sky. The air was crisp and refreshing and lovely on my skin. I had released the need to be well cared for by someone who was not able or available to do so. I began to protect my own inner, sacred core. A lesson I continue to learn how to do again and again. I went home and I held my baby. I offered my breast and fed this little child. I softened around my broken and empty places in complete trust that they'd be perfectly filled in divine timing. And divine timing and provision have never failed me yet.

## Know Yourself

So the paradox is that we need to be willing to keep open spaces in our lives until the right relationships come but we also need to reach out in courage and take chances to receive intimacy, love, and help from others. Breaking the isolation is very difficult for many of us. We have wounded mothers all over the place who don't have critical maternal networks in place and are trying to do this on their own. It's crucial, though, as you begin to reach out and fill your need for authentic connections to get clear on how you're best supported and what does (and doesn't) work for you.

Case in point: Playgroups with toddlers are quite possibly the most painful experiences I've had to endure. I know for many moms this is an amazing opportunity for connection and they've met some of their best friends through early playgroups. But, for me, this was just not my scene. I remember one day in particular, Jackson was climbing the book case in this lovely woman's living room and Madelyn, still an infant, was refusing the bottle I had brought for her. My boobs were so full and aching with milk that I had to excuse myself and go into the bathroom, and while balancing her on my knees, I pumped with my travel pump just to relieve the pain. Outside the closed door I could hear Jackson start to cry in the other room. On top of it all, I was desperately trying to keep my voice calm and keep up a conversation through the door, reminding Jackson I'd be right out and not to climb anything. I can assure you I left far more depleted than I walked in that afternoon. For a while, even though I knew I needed connection, I just didn't know where to look to find it in ways that worked for me. It's so important to honor where you are and who you are. These inner hut relationships don't have to look like what works for other people. Many times it's simply trial and error, exploring what groups and communities feel right to you.

## When It Looks Different Than You Expect

It's also a good idea to look at what's already right in front of you. It may be an amazing relationship that just doesn't look like what you expect it to. When I was pregnant with Jackson, none of my closest girlfriends at the time were local or were moms. So I joined a prenatal yoga class partly for my own wellbeing and partly to see if I could connect with other soon-to-be moms in the area. I can remember the group was full of lovely women, but many of them were pregnant with their second or third children, tired, and already booked with busy schedules and no connections really took off for me. At about the same time I reconnected with an old friend, Jessica, who I'd gone to elementary and middle school with years ago. She was also pregnant, with her second, and it was great to catch up with her.

Now, Jessica and I from most angles are opposites. I've always loved her, but our lives just went in different directions after high school. My idea of a vacation was a weeklong backpacking trip into the mountains, and being dirty without a shower was her idea of a nightmare. But underneath we were so aligned. She has one of the biggest hearts of any person I know … generous, committed, and always thinking of others. And so real. She was one of the first people I ever talked to who didn't try and sugar coat all the crazy paradoxes you feel as a mother. So when I was a wreck because I couldn't calm my colicky baby, or the sling wearing wasn't working, or the breastfeeding was so damn painful I cried through all the feedings, or when I felt nauseous in fear over all the things I read on the Internet that could go wrong with my newborn … she was my rock. Jessica would call me every single day. I didn't talk to my mother every day. In fact, I've never really been a phone call kind of friend. But Jessica saw how hurting I was and she was not going to let me go. Even though my tendency was to crawl into a hole with how hard it all felt, she refused to let me be in there alone. She climbed her way into the cave with me some days just so I could feel someone else next to me. It can still bring me to tears to know the depth of her commitment to me and our friendship. As you begin to assess the circle of people around you be sure not to miss out on some of the most treasured members of your inner hut just because they don't look like what you thought they'd look like. Consider the true nature of your relationships and how they impact your own wellbeing and life.

## Messiness Is Part of the Deal

Finally, relationships are messy. It can feel like it's better to go without them than to risk feeling hurt or let down. I think being brought to my knees in neediness was the greatest blessing of all because it required me to break through the falsehood of believing I could do it all myself and drove me to connection, even when it felt awkward and uncomfortable. And relationships can feel awkward and uncomfortable. Just because I knew finding the right support networks was essential, didn't mean it happened overnight or that I didn't have a number of disappointments and wrong turns along the way. I'm still building my inner circle, but I'm light years ahead of where I was as a new mother. I'm coming to understand the process of staying open to authentic connection and to receiving the gift of meaningful relationships in my life.

Cultivating Authentic Connections in your life and building your inner hut circle is about mastering the art of boundaries and access within relationships. You need both. But often we get these things utterly backward. We hedge ourselves from true intimacy and connection (which comes with vulnerability) and we give free access to people who, time and time again, leave us feeling depleted and even more isolated—all in the name of trying to fit into social norms and expectations. We can spend our time trying to search out new relationships that look like the shiny-happy-easy ones we dream about in our heads while we don't see the real, authentic, and messy ones right in front of us. Even your inner hut connections will feel messy sometimes—human relationships are—but when we can start seeing the gifts we gain within these relationships we're more likely to invest in growing them deep and strong. Here's a review of the tools we explored to build up the core essential of Authentic Connections in our lives.

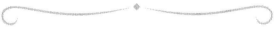

## Authentic Connections Tool Box

- *Take stock of who you let into your inner hut circle and consider if they are edifying or draining*

- *Consider the three types of Inner Hut connections and whether you have people in your life that fill them: Soul–Sisters, Mentors, and Visionaries*

- *Create clear and strong boundaries between relationships that feel unaligned with who you are and who you're becoming ... allow empty spaces rather than keeping people in your life who are unworthy to be close to you*

- *Get to know how you best need and want to be supported*

- *Consider if you're overlooking key relationships that already exist in your life because they look different than you imagined they'd look*

- *Be open to the messiness of relationships—extend grace to others in ways you'd want grace extended to you*

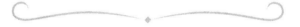

# Chapter 9

# Sacred Schedules

This whole book we've been talking about powerful ways we can replenish and restore our wellbeing so we radiate fullness from within. But these seven core essentials, and all the tools that go along with them, are useless if we don't take back our time and elevate our wellbeing to priority status in our schedules. The way you spend your time is the way you spend your life. There's a huge difference between having the information in your head and practicing it in your life. It takes a fierce commitment to break through the patterns of already established habits in our lives and make room for new habits to be born. That's why we need to see our schedules as sacred, because our schedules are really the way in which we spend our time, our choices, and our focus … and so they make up what becomes of our lives.

## The Wise Woman and the Warrior

To make this kind of course correction, both the wise woman and the warrior need to rise within us. The wise woman within each of us knows when life's not going well and begins to seek out true wisdom. She shifts inwardly and asks the hard questions. She seeks upwardly and asks for guidance and insight. She seeks the counsel of others through conversations and books. She analyzes what's working and not working in her life. She asks questions and begins to gain clarity. This is all a crucial and important part of the process of change. The wise woman must surface first before real change can happen in our lives.

But for a long time in my life, I would find myself stuck in the wise woman part of the change journey. I found myself writing the same things over and over again in my journal, knowing in my heart what wasn't working, but waking up every day to the same patterns, the same routine, the same dullness and discontent. Something else is needed if wisdom is going to make any real difference in our lives. The "Warrior" needs to rise up. Because in today's society, growing your own self into the person you want to be … and developing into the mother you need to be for your children requires both wise insight and a willingness to fight for the life you want. In order to shift into a life that is deeply aligned from the inside out, that generates inner peace and contentment, that exudes happiness and confidence, you must be willing to fight for it. To protect yourself and your family from all the influences and noise and confusion coming at you from every side. To shield against the distractions that keep you in an A.D.D. state of scattered thoughts and impulsive decisions.

It's the tag team of wise woman and warrior that needs to rise up in you when you're really ready to become the woman you long to be—a woman comfortable in your own skin again and equipped to live the life you were called to. In short, the warrior has the courage and commitment to make the changes necessary to align her outer life with her inner life. She takes back sovereignty of her time, thoughts, and choices so the life she desires becomes the life she lives. And so it was crucial that I end this book with strategies on how to make these seven core essentials a regular, habitual part of our lives—because only then can they actually replenish us and provide the radiant calm and true vitality that we want.

# How to Begin

It was very early in the morning. My small, battery powered alarm clock woke me at 4:00 am to a silent world around me. I was in an unfamiliar, small bed in a little room off the kitchen of my host family's home in Guatemala. I was living, volunteering, and studying here for a couple months one summer during college. I got dressed quickly and grabbed the cheese sandwich and banana they'd left me on the kitchen table and hopped into a van waiting outside the front door to join the other students planning to hike Santa Maria with me.

We arrived at the foot of the volcano. While the stars were still bright and pulsing in the dark sky and we began our ascent. The hike would take hours, so we began early in order to make it to the top and back home by dinner time. We followed the thin dirt path carved into the side of the volcano, traversing our way back and forth through stretches of grassy wildflowers and rocky outcroppings. About three hours into the hike, we entered the stretch of mountain where the clouds hung low and you could hike in and through different cloud clusters for a while. This was where I saw my first holy man.

About halfway up the ascent, I began seeing little parts of the mountain wall carved out just enough that someone could jimmy themselves into the small indent and allow others to pass by on the trail. At first, I assumed these little carved out areas were there in case someone needed to rest or was injured, so they could find a place to sit while others hiked by. But soon I learned the holy men of the community used these outcroppings as places to pause, burn incense, read their holy books, and pray as they hiked their way to the peak. Our guide told us that the priests and healers of the village always hiked the local mountains during their prayer times. What occurred to me was these holy men were not so much closer to God as they prayed higher and higher up the mountain, but rather they were further away from the world. And when we give ourselves the space to be further away from the world and the world's needs and demands, we can more easily focus on that which is most important and true.

Sometimes we need to create a little distance, slow down the pace from the frenetic rush of our lives in order to recreate a life that's congruent with what's most important to us. I was once on a walk at trail near my home. My mind was racing with so many stressful thoughts, and I was rushing my way through the path like a speed-walker. I remember saying to God in my head, "How do I just slow down a little?" And I felt him say to me, "How do you slow down, Lisa? ... Stop walking so fast." I just stood there with a half smile on my face realizing how ridiculous it was that I was practically running through this walk wondering why my mind couldn't calm down. So I found a downed log and sat by the creek and let my body lead the way of calming my mind. I just took in the world around me and the thoughts settled down in accord.   My life is very full, as I'm sure is yours. What I've came to understand along the way is there's a difference between busyness and fullness. When I tip the scale from fullness to busyness, the quality of my life begins to suffer.

## Fence Posts Fixes

Imagine a long wooden fence post of the Old West kind with short vertical wooden posts holding up long stretches of horizontal posts. The vertical posts are your practices of self care. They're the tools that are part of your life which keep your seven core essentials of wellbeing nourished and nurtured. The horizontal stretches of fence are your life—your day to day living, your relationships, your responsibilities, your to-do lists … everything that's "on your plate." The heavier the horizontal posts become, the closer the vertical posts need to be. You need more vertical posts placed in your life when your life is more intense, more demanding, when more is required of you to give at a higher level. The vertical posts are what give the horizontal posts their strength. When you feel the sway and bend of the horizontal posts in your life, you know you need to place more vertical posts more often into your life.

So the vertical posts (which make up the whole of your self-care practice) are a mixture of two types of posts. First there are the established posts you put into your life as habits of your wellbeing and that you can always depend upon to be there at certain intervals, every day, every week, or every month. I call this your non-negotiable self care practices, the bare minimum you will commit to on a daily, weekly or monthly basis because you know this is what you need to feel your best.

Then, there are the flexible posts that you can grab and put in place when you need them in the moment or when you know there's a challenging stretch ahead. Remember, many of the tools we've talk about throughout this book can be brought in with minimal effort. You can take a few minutes for a deep, cleansing breath, or grab a calming food, or sooth your nervous system with a mini neck massage, or call a dear friend who will listen and laugh and love you up, or take out your journal and write out a messy, heart-wrenching prayer to God, or take a ten minute walk outside to clear your mind. These are all posts available to you when the weight of life feels intense to hold. This isn't a prescription, it's a process. There are times when we can go further without as many vertical posts; there are times when they need to be lined up every six inches. The important thing is to get used to checking into your life and responding to your needs before you get to empty or past the breaking point.

You allow the needs of your life to dictate how often and which posts to put into place. As you get better and better at tuning in to your own needs you'll find this process more and more fluid. I can now look forward to my month, assess my home life and work life needs, and schedule in the supports that will help me meet those needs without sacrificing my core wellbeing. I can also reach out for help and let those close to me know when I'll need extra support and love. Another way I know when more vertical posts need to be put in place is when I start to feel a lack of "fruits" in my life.

## Lead by Fruits

In nature, fruits are the gifts that plants give to the world. And you can tell the nature of the plant's health by the kind of fruit it bears. In our lives, fruits are the expressions of how well we are doing on the inside. To understand how fruits show up for you, imagine you're experiencing complete and vibrant health in a certain area of your life. For example, let's take a healthy body. If my body was experiencing vibrant health, what would that feel like to me? When my body is truly healthy, I feel strong, light, energized, and flexible. So strong, light, energized, and flexible, for me, are the fruits of a healthy body. When my body begins to feel heavy, congested, lethargic, or stiff—I know I need to adjust something. I can look to the core essentials and consider which may need more attention.

Here are some more examples of fruits in other core areas of our whole-person wellbeing. (I'm sharing the fruits that are true for me. Work through these examples and consider for yourself what the fruits are for you.) The fruits of my healthy mind are clarity, focus, active learning, and creative problem solving. When one or more of these fruits aren't present in my life, I know I need to support myself a little more to keep my mind healthy and active. The fruits of my healthy mood are calmness, happiness, positivity, and feeling emotionally grounded when life gets challenging. When I find myself vacillating between mood swings and extremes, I know I need some more support in caring for my emotional health. The fruits of my healthy spirit are a sense of knowing all is well and trusting I'm perfectly provided for, feeling grace toward myself and others, and a desire to spread the love I'm feeling inside to those around me. When I'm well plugged into my Creator, this is the natural outpouring of my heart. When I get impatient, anxious, or closed off from those I love, it's clear I need more supports in feeding my spiritual health.

Sounds easy, right? It is, but only once it becomes a habit. The part that requires work (which it does) is recreating these habits of wellbeing in your life. But it's such worthy work and it pays back in dividends every time. So, in the beginning, if you've neglected your own health and well being for a while, making the changes necessary to feel the fruits of a healthy body may take a bit longer, they may require multiple ways to nourish and care for your body. But every time you layer in another self-care practice, you move in the direction of healing and the fruits will bear in the right time. After a while you start to notice your own "danger zones" when you no longer are experiencing the fruits of wellness in your life—or when the "anti-fruits" are starting to show up. Sometimes I can catch an anti-fruit faster than the lack of a fruit. For example, sometimes I don't realize my lack of focus until I'm keenly aware of how scattered my mind feels—two sides of the same coin. But if you have certain "anti-fruits" that you tend to experience when your tank is getting dangerously low, it's good to become aware of them and allow them to signal the need to make some simple, fast changes to support yourself.

# Making Space, One Fence Post at a Time

Motherhood often asks us to embrace the messiness in order to find the clarity. So I've found the only way is to begin is by working on one fence post at a time. Once I got clear on the one fence post of support I was going to bring into my life, I would intentionally make changes to my schedule in order to give that new habit space to take root. One core essential at a time became a non-negotiable priority for me and the rest of my life needed to make small adjustments and shifts in order to allow it to come in. In my journey, I started with Restorative Rest. I made the commitment to prioritize a simple thirty minute evening routine and early bedtime. I clung to it like a warrior (or like a drowning person). I like to see myself as a warrior now fighting for my own wellbeing, but it felt more like an exhausted person stranded at sea, clinging to whatever floating pieces of wood I could grab. So I chose one fence post and I cleared my plate and opened up my schedule so restorative rest had room to root and become a habit of wellbeing. I had to rethink work I had been delegating into the late evening hours; I had to rethink the house chores I did after the kids went to sleep. I had to rethink the time I spent spacing out on the computer. It didn't feel easy to clear that space in my life, but I knew I had to cross the threshold between wanting change and committing to change. That, of course, made all the difference.

You'll find that sometimes the most miraculous of things happen when you make one small choice for your own wellbeing. That one choice to fiercely protect my sleep ended up naturally rearranging many other things in my life. Like a Rubik's cube, that one adjustment shifted how I prioritized time during the day to get my work complete—and it allowed me the grace to set more appropriate goals for myself around what I wanted to accomplish through my work during this season of my life.

It changed how I handled the bedtime routine with my kids, because now it was also my bedtime routine and I was clear and consistent with it, which benefited all of us. I began to wake with a radically different level of energy and clarity (even though I was still being woken up multiple times a night by my little ones). Going to bed earlier was making a huge difference in my capacity to manage the ups and downs of my day.

## How to Choose Where to Start

If you find yourself where I did a couple years ago, where so many areas of your wellbeing need to be refilled, you have no idea where to start, I get it. Truly, I do. And you're not alone. Chronic depletion muddles and confuses the next right step. It masks as perfection and convinces you things are so broken, that small positive shifts couldn't possibly make a difference. When we're already feeling maxed out and overwhelmed reading a book on self care can feel more head-spinning than heart-soothing. So if you're experiencing that sense of inner shut down, here's an exercise that'll help narrow down a first step.

## The Core Essentials Circle

Look at the circle below and either mark this paper or re-draw it on a separate piece of paper. Each spike in the circle represents one of the seven core essentials of your wellbeing. The place on each line at the very center, where all spokes come together, means completely unsatisfied and the place on each line that touches the edge of the circle means completely satisfied.[17]

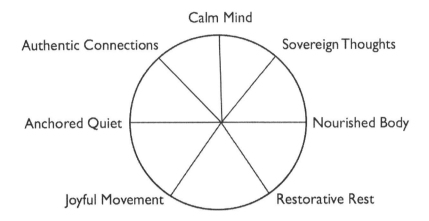

The Core Essentials Circle

You're going to consider each core essential in turn and ask yourself, "How am I doing in this area of my wellbeing?" Now put a dot somewhere along the line for each core essential. If you're feeling extremely satisfied, strong and vital in that area, put a dot where the line touches the outer edge of the circle. If you're feeling extremely dissatisfied, neglected or depleted in that area, put a dot where the line touches the center. Or if you are feeling somewhere in between those extremes put a dot approximately where you feel you land for each core essential.

Now you can connect your dots and assess your personal Core Essentials Circle. The places which are most collapsed are the areas that need your attention first. Consider choosing one of these core essentials to begin with and take it one small step at a time. And truly, that's all you need to focus on—one positive step at a time. Once you work through the Circle of Core Essentials Exercise, decide on one core essential and then one tool or strategy that will support it and start there. You can never predict the impact or changes one small act of caring will have in your life right now, so don't worry about the steps ahead. Just begin with one good and loving act of self-care right now.

# Epilogue

One afternoon when I was writing this book in my office, my daughter brought me a picture she had drawn from her preschool class. It was a bright sun, a cloud with rain coming down, and swirls of air in the sky. She also colored brown earth and green grass with a bright orange flower in the middle. She handed it to me and asked, "Mom, do you know what a flower needs to grow?" And before I could finish my smile, she informed me that it needs four things in order to grow like it's meant to: sunlight, water, soil, and air. I couldn't help but think this little diagram captured exactly what I was trying to say in fifty-thousand words with my book.

## What does a mama need to grow?

What does a mama need to grow? What are the raw materials we need intricately woven into our days in order to live vibrant and healthy lives? To be fully growing, engaged and happy women? To show up as our best selves as we live, love, and mother in our everyday lives?

In short, how do we stop treading water long enough in order to catch our breath and learn different ways of living so we show up as our best and brightest selves? In this book we explored seven core essentials to our wellbeing. Each, like a hose filling a pool, can contribute to the rising waters without being on full blast. Each can offer a trickle and the plastic balls of our wellbeing will all rise together.

I want to end by sharing a visual meditation that I use when I need to remind myself why this work is so important and why filling the well is non-negotiable as I seek to become the best version of myself in the world—the best woman, wife, and mother I can be. As you read this next section, soften your eyes, remove distracting noises, and relax into your soft body and fluid breath. Wrap these words with images in your mind and let them settle deep into your thoughts. Then spend a few minutes in quiet reflection, perhaps even journaling, as you feel fully into the vibrant, whole and healthy woman you're becoming.

## Sacred Core Imagery

Envision within the center of your body an energy rod. I imagine mine as a long rod shape down the center of my torso, but perhaps your is a star, or a ball. Just feel your energy core within you and allow whatever shape, color, feel it takes to be perfect. Focus softly on this glowing, rippling energy center within you and imagine it spilling over like a waterfall or gurgling hot spring out into the world around you in color and radiance. Imagine a bright, radiant light from the center of your body flowing out into the world around you.

Imagine your family standing near you (bring them near in your mind's eye: your spouse, your children, your loved ones). Imagine they are bathed playfully and beautifully in this light. Covered in its radiance and warmth. There is plenty. There is more than enough. There is abundance of this beautiful light. When we're living from a full well, we are nourishing and protecting our inner core—our inner life force. The gift of God's light living in us. You protect and replenish your sacred core by the feeding and care of your body, heart, mind, and soul. You enlarge the capacity of your spirit to receive this inner light by being a good steward of your whole person and keeping yourself well and cared for.

Your core life energy is filled and radiating. From that place you have natural overflow—you have ripples of your life energy that can spill over and give to those you love from an abundant place. From that connected place you're generous and patient. You're quick to smile and serve. You're playful and light. You're full of confidence and insight. You're content and happy. I want you to see the direction of the energy that is flowing and abundant as running in a vertical manner—it runs down into deep roots of self care, self kindness, self nurture ... and it runs up and over into service and generosity and outward energy in the world. Sit in this place and truly feel yourself in this place. Imagine yourself interacting with your children, with our spouse, in your home, in our community.

This feels so different than the model most of us experience of giving in our day to day life as mothers. When you are ready to shift out of this meditation, consider what your life energy looks like when it's tapped out and drained. When you feel exhausted and exasperated. When there's depletion. Imagine your energy during these times as spread horizontally. No roots. Nothing protecting it or replenishing it. Stretched thin across too far of a range. Instead of sourcing from a full and vibrant center space within you, it's scattered and weak.

What we need to learn to do is protect our life energy and to direct it so that it stays strong and anchored. Fortress it so that it can establish deep roots and be directed upward and outward, rather than siphoned and squandered. And that's what the gift of tending to the core essentials does for us. They give us ground under our feet so we don't need to tread breathless everyday—

going through the motions and getting through the day. Instead, when the fundamentals are taken care of, we can begin to use our tremendous gifts of calm and vitality to radiate outward and bless those we love most in our lives. We get to give generous gifts of love and service. And we get to experience the profound gift of living out our best lives and shining our brightest lights during our most important years.

# References

1. Drowning Doesn't Look Like Drowning by Mario Vittone: http://mariovittone.com/2010/05/154/

2. Donna Eden: http://innersource.net/em/about/donna-eden.html

3. A Potential Natural Treatment for Attention-Deficit/Hyperactivity Disorder: Evidence From a National Study : http://www.ncbi.nlm.nih.gov/pmc/articles/PMC1448497/

4. How Stress Influences Disease: Carnegie Mellon Study Reveals Inflammation as the Culprit : http://www.cmu.edu/news/stories/archives/2012/april/april2_stressdisease.html

5. "You are a soul. You have a body." -George MacDonald: http://mereorthodoxy.com/you-dont-have-a-soul-cs-lewis-never-said-it/

6. MAPP Gathering interview with Jennifer Louden: http://www.mappgathering.com/jennifer-louden/

7. Medina, John J. 2009 Brain Rules Pear Press

8. MAPP Gathering interview with Tsh Oxenreider: http://www.mappgathering.com/tsh-oxenreider/

9. Omvana app: http://www.omvana.com/

10. Effects of interruptions, length of time and error rates: Ramsey, NF et al (2003) Neurophysiological factors in human information processing capacity 127: 517 - 525

11. Father Thomas Keating and the Contemplative Movement: http://www.contemplativeoutreach.org/fr-thomas-keating

12. Binaural research: http://www.monroeinstitute.org/research/the-history-of-research-at-the-monroe-institute

13. Mondo Beyondo course: http://www.mondobeyondo.org/

14. Ann Voskamp: http://www.aholyexperience.com/

15. Research on mirror neurons: http://greatergood.berkeley.edu/article/item/do_mirror_neurons_give_empathy

16. Real Women Talking website: http://realwomentalkingnow.com/

17. Circle of Core Essentials was inspired by Circle of Life - an exercise I learned while studying at the Institute for Integrative Nutrition: http://www.integrativenutrition.com/

# Gratitude

Writing this book has been an incredible (and intense) journey of processing my own story of motherhood so far. I'm left with a heart flooded over in gratitude for the amazing little beings I get to call my children and who teach me daily what it really means to love in this world.

And for Michael, the one I walk hand in hand, heart in heart, with through all the twists and turns of this great adventure. It's no overstatement to say without you this book simply could not have happened. Beyond believing in me and supporting me ... you stepped up and shouldered the additional weight of our lives in order to make sure I keep the passion-fire burning inside me for the work I do through WellGrounded Life. I cannot find adequate words to describe the treasure I have in you. I love you, honey.

I'm grateful that, regardless of my resistance, God led me back to New Jersey to raise my littles among the circle of my first inner hut, my mother and sister. I'm grateful to have you each in my life and to watch my own children's lives become richer because you love them.

I'm indebted to the tremendously huge-hearted and wildly skilled Bren who came alongside me a couple years ago and said,

"I need to work for you." Beyond the love and talent she's poured into WellGrounded Life, she's also become one of my dearest friends and biggest cheerleaders. Bren: I thank God daily for you. And for Donna, our newest team member who's so seamlessly fit into our team, I can hardly remember a time when you weren't a part of us. It's like a double rainbow I gaze at each day working with you both.

A special word of love and gratitude for Shelly, my sister-soul friend, who, I'm convinced, is part angel walking among us, for seeing me and holding me with such love, gentleness, and kindness, I feel strengthened simply by knowing you're in my world. And for Jessica, who's commitment to our friendship has never faded over decades—what a thrill to come full circle and raise our children together. For Kristin, who so generously gives of her precious time, wise insight and grace-filled care, spending hours with me on the phone, holding my hand (and heart) as I muddle through this messy road of mothering—thank you, dear friend.

For all the mothers in the WellGrounded Life community—who've been part of my courses and who've trusted me as their coach—it's such a tremendous honor to know you and journey beside you for a while. And for those in my course communities who've become for each other beacons of grace and strength, wisdom and love—I'm indebted in gratitude for who you are and the gift you give by showing up and sharing yourselves with each other. If there's one thing I'm sure of, what heals a mama most is to be seen, cared for and part of a loving, grace-drenched community. And that's what each of the women who are part of WellGrounded Life has made this place to be.

# About the Author

Lisa Grace Byrne is an author, speaker, teacher and trusted authority on vitality and wellbeing for mothers. She's the founder of WellGrounded Life an exceptional community where she teaches courses, workshops and classes that help mothers live self-connected, healthy, and vibrant lives.

Lisa's degrees are from Cal Poly State University in Biochemistry with an emphasis in Nutrition and Metabolism and from Boston University where she holds a Masters in Public Health. She's a Certified Holistic Health Counselor through the Institute for Integrative Nutrition and Columbia University. Lisa lives in New Jersey with her three children, husband and 110 pound yellow lab.

Learn more about her work and resources at www.WellGroundedLife.com

# An Invitation…
## The WellGrounded Life Community

I began this work with mothers four years ago when I felt I was drowning in my own life. I simply reached out a hand believing that if I needed help so desperately, perhaps another mom out there needed help too. What I didn't expect was the outpouring of hands that reached back to grab mine. I didn't expect the simple movement of reaching out, just a little, would impact my own wellbeing so profoundly. I didn't realize the power of many hands grasped together in grace-filled, loving intention to care for each other and support each other toward getting back on dry land. It's been a wonder for me to behold. If you haven't been connected to my online community at WellGrounded Life, I invite you with my whole heart to come and explore what we have to offer and the ways in which we serve mothers all over the world.

Here are some ways to get connected.

### Say Hello

- I have a twitter account (www.twitter.com/wellgrounded), but I'm much more active on Facebook. You can connect

to the WellGrounded Life Facebook page here: www.facebook.com/wellgrounded.
- Pinterest is getting rather addicting these days, hop over to connect with us there. (http://pinterest.com/wellgroundedlif/)
- Email our team with any insights, questions, or feedback at team@wellgroundedlife.com

## Free Stuff

- We've got gifts for you! To enhance your experience with this book, I've put together a virtual bonus pack ready for immediate download. Go to: www.WellGroundedLife.com/replenishbonus

## Workshops and Courses

By far the best way to tap into the gold of WellGrounded Life's offerings is through taking a workshop, class or course with me. Below are a sampling of the courses we offer and the ways to learn more.

- **Teach Your Life to be Extraordinary**
  Discover how to bring purpose and passion into your life as a modern mother without compromising your family. In this course, you'll design the layout of your "Life Garden." We'll take a bird's eye view of your life as it is now and then dream of where you want to grow. We'll hone in on the 5 P's of an extraordinary life—purpose, passion, path of service, priorities and prosperity—and explore how to realign your outer life to match your inner heart. Together we'll carve out room for joy to grow through reflection, assessment and planning of how you spend your precious time and energy.

- **Designed for Wellness**

  This is a healthy eating, vibrant living course for busy moms. It equips you to get healthy, fresh, whole foods into you and your family's diet without chaining you to the kitchen for hours of prep work. It's my signature course because it lays the foundation of high level wellness through food and nutrition.

- **Harmonize Your Hormones**

  Balance your hormones for a calm, productive, energized life. In this course, we tend our root system which is our hormonal health and balance. Harmonize Your Hormones fine tunes your inner hormonal balance through deeply restorative self care practices, targeted nutrition, mind-body work, herbal supports, self examination and energetic work.

- **Cleanse Your Life**

  Whole Body-Whole Life Cleanse and Detox. Finally, there comes a time in all of our gardens when a good weeding is necessary. Cleanse Your Life is a clearing out of the gunk that's keeping your systems clogged, your mind sluggish and your home messy. It focuses on detoxifying and cleansing your body, yourself care products, your environment, your kitchen, your pantry and your home hot spots. Just like intense bouts of weeding, this course is meant to build momentum to take you from a healthy living funk to a high energy gallop.

To learn more about these courses, visit
www.WellGroundedLife.com/all-courses/